MIDM000289259

Integrating Physical Activity Into Cancer Care:
An Evidence-Based Approach

Edited by
Lisa Marie Bernardo, PhD, MPH, RN, CEP, CCET
Betsy J. Becker, PT, DPT, CLT-LANA

Oncology Nursing Society
Pittsburgh, Pennsylvania

ONS Publications Department
Publisher and Director of Publications: William A. Tony, BA, CQIA
Managing Editor: Lisa M. George, BA
Assistant Managing Editor: Amy Nicoletti, BA, JD
Acquisitions Editor: John Zaphyr, BA, MEd
Copy Editors: Vanessa Kattouf, BA, Andrew Petyak, BA
Graphic Designer: Dany Sjoen
Editorial Assistant: Judy Holmes

Library of Congress Cataloging-in-Publication Data
Names: Bernardo, Lisa Marie, editor. | Becker, Betsy J., editor. | Oncology
    Nursing Society, issuing body.
Title: Integrating physical activity into cancer care : an evidence-based
    approach / edited by Lisa Marie Bernardo, Betsy J. Becker.
Description: Pittsburgh, Pennsylvania : Oncology Nursing Society, [2016] |
    Includes bibliographical references and index.
Identifiers: LCCN 2016034544 | ISBN 9781935864912
Subjects: | MESH: Neoplasms--therapy | Exercise Therapy--methods | Motor
    Activity | Physical Therapy Modalities | Evidence-Based Practice | Nurses'
    Instruction
Classification: LCC RC271.P44 | NLM QZ 266 | DDC 616.99/4062--dc23 LC record available at https://lccn.
    loc.gov/2016034544

Publisher's Note
This book is published by the Oncology Nursing Society (ONS). ONS neither represents nor guarantees that the practices described herein will, if followed, ensure safe and effective patient care. The recommendations contained in this book reflect ONS's judgment regarding the state of general knowledge and practice in the field as of the date of publication. The recommendations may not be appropriate for use in all circumstances. Those who use this book should make their own determinations regarding specific safe and appropriate patient care practices, taking into account the personnel, equipment, and practices available at the hospital or other facility at which they are located. The editors and publisher cannot be held responsible for any liability incurred as a consequence from the use or application of any of the contents of this book. Figures and tables are used as examples only. They are not meant to be all-inclusive, nor do they represent endorsement of any particular institution by ONS. Mention of specific products and opinions related to those products do not indicate or imply endorsement by ONS. Websites mentioned are provided for information only; the hosts are responsible for their own content and availability. Unless otherwise indicated, dollar amounts reflect U.S. dollars.

ONS publications are originally published in English. Publishers wishing to translate ONS publications must contact ONS about licensing arrangements. ONS publications cannot be translated without obtaining written permission from ONS. (Individual tables and figures that are reprinted or adapted require additional permission from the original source.) Because translations from English may not always be accurate or precise, ONS disclaims any responsibility for inaccuracies in words or meaning that may occur as a result of the translation. Readers relying on precise information should check the original English version.

Printed in the United States of America

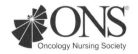

Innovation • Excellence • Advocacy

Contributors

Editors

Lisa Marie Bernardo, PhD, MPH, RN, CEP, CCET
Managing Member
The Pilates Center, LLC
Gibsonia, Pennsylvania
Nursing Research Consultant
Excela Health
Greensburg, Pennsylvania

Betsy J. Becker, PT, DPT, CLT-LANA
Assistant Professor, Division of Physical
 Therapy Education
College of Allied Health Professions
University of Nebraska Medical Center
Omaha, Nebraska
*Chapter 5. Assessing Readiness for
Physical Activity; Chapter 6. Assessing
Readiness for Physical Activity: Physical
Considerations; Chapter 7. Evaluating
Tolerance and Adherence to Physical
Activity; Chapter 15. Support Groups and
Resources*

Authors

Catherine M. Bender, PhD, RN, FAAN
Professor, Nursing and Clinical and
 Translational Science Institute
Nancy Glunt Hoffman Endowed Chair
 in Oncology Nursing
University of Pittsburgh School of
 Nursing
Pittsburgh, Pennsylvania
*Chapter 9. Physical Activity for Cognitive
Functioning*

Ann M. Berger, PhD, APRN, AOCNS®, FAAN
Professor and Dorothy Hodges Olson
 Endowed Chair
Advanced Practice Nurse
University of Nebraska Medical Center
Omaha, Nebraska
*Chapter 11. Physical Activity for Promot-
ing Sleep*

Kerry S. Courneya, PhD
Professor and Canada Research Chair
Faculty of Physical Education and
    Recreation
University of Alberta
Edmonton, Alberta, Canada
*Chapter 2. Physical Activity and Cancer
Survival; Chapter 14. Physical Activity and
Cancer Survival: Future Directions*

**Justin C. Deskovich, DPT, MPT, OCS,
    SCS, DAC, CSCS, COMT, FAAOMPT,
    FMS Cert.**
Doctor of Physical Therapy and
    Co-Owner
Back 2 Action Physical Therapy
Farmington, Pennsylvania
Managing Physical Therapist
Orthopedic and Sports Physical
    Therapy Associates, Inc.
Morgantown, West Virginia
*Chapter 10. Physical Activity for Cancer-
Related Pain*

Katrina Fetter, MSN, RN, OCN®
Oncology Clinical Educator
Lancaster General Health/Penn Medicine
Lancaster, Pennsylvania
*Chapter 3. Promoting Physical Activity for
Cancer Survivors*

Jean Godfroy, RN, BSN, CBCN®, OCN®
Clinical Nurse Coordinator, Breast
    Program
Froedtert Hospital
Milwaukee, Wisconsin
*Chapter 8. Physical Activity for Cancer-
Related Fatigue*

Julie Griffie, RN, MSN, AOCN®
Clinical Nurse Specialist
Froedtert Hospital
Milwaukee, Wisconsin
*Chapter 8. Physical Activity for Cancer-
Related Fatigue*

Olivia Huffman, PT, DPT
Physical Therapist
Quantum Health Professionals
Kansas City, Kansas
*Chapter 15. Support Groups and
Resources*

Jeannette Q. Lee, PT, PhD
Assistant Professor
University of California, San Francisco/
    San Francisco State University Grad-
    uate Program in Physical Therapy
San Francisco, California
*Chapter 4. FITT Principle for Physical
Activity*

Amy J. Litterini, PT, DPT
Assistant Clinical Professor, Depart-
    ment of Physical Therapy
University of New England
Portland, Maine
*Chapter 12. Physical Activity for Chronic
Cancer-Related Conditions; Chapter 13.
Physical Activity for Metastatic and End-
of-Life Conditions*

**Ellyn E. Matthews, PhD, RN, AOCNS®,
    CBSM, FAAN**
Associate Professor and Elizabeth
    Stanley Cooper Endowed Chair in
    Oncology Nursing
University of Arkansas for Medical
    Sciences
Little Rock, Arkansas
*Chapter 11. Physical Activity for Promot-
ing Sleep*

Kelly McCormick, PT, DPT
Physical Therapist
Imua Physical Therapy
Maui, Hawaii
*Chapter 15. Support Groups and
Resources*

Andria R. Morielli, MSc
PhD student
Faculty of Physical Education and
    Recreation
University of Alberta
Edmonton, Alberta, Canada
*Chapter 2. Physical Activity and Cancer
Survival; Chapter 14. Physical Activity and
Cancer Survival: Future Directions*

Alaina Newell, PT, DPT, WCS, CLT-LANA
Oncology and Women's Health Physical Therapy Specialist
Oncology Rehab
Centennial, Colorado
Chapter 5. Assessing Readiness for Physical Activity; Chapter 6. Assessing Readiness for Physical Activity: Physical Considerations; Chapter 7. Evaluating Tolerance and Adherence to Physical Activity

Kathryn E. Tasillo, PT, DPT
Lead Medical Surgical Therapist
Carolinas Medical Center
Carolinas HealthCare System
Charlotte, North Carolina
Chapter 1. Overview

Kara Tischer, PT, DPT
Physical Therapist
Quantum Health Professionals
Omaha, Nebraska
Chapter 15. Support Groups and Resources

Linda Trinh, PhD
Assistant Professor
Department of Kinesiology and Community Health
University of Illinois at Urbana–Champaign
Urbana, Illinois
Chapter 2. Physical Activity and Cancer Survival; Chapter 14. Physical Activity and Cancer Survival: Future Directions

Frances Westlake, PT, DPT, NCS
Neuro-Vestibular Physical Therapist
Oncology Rehab
Centennial, Colorado
Chapter 5. Assessing Readiness for Physical Activity; Chapter 6. Assessing Readiness for Physical Activity: Physical Considerations; Chapter 7. Evaluating Tolerance and Adherence to Physical Activity

Disclosure

Editors and authors of books and guidelines provided by the Oncology Nursing Society are expected to disclose to the readers any significant financial interest or other relationships with the manufacturer(s) of any commercial products.

A vested interest may be considered to exist if a contributor is affiliated with or has a financial interest in commercial organizations that may have a direct or indirect interest in the subject matter. A "financial interest" may include, but is not limited to, being a shareholder in the organization; being an employee of the commercial organization; serving on an organization's speakers bureau; or receiving research funding from the organization. An "affiliation" may be holding a position on an advisory board or some other role of benefit to the commercial organization. Vested interest statements appear in the front matter for each publication.

Contributors are expected to disclose any unlabeled or investigational use of products discussed in their content. This information is acknowledged solely for the information of the readers.

The contributors provided the following disclosure and vested interest information:
Betsy J. Becker, PT, DPT, CLT-LANA: University of Nebraska Medical Center, Next Step Cancer Recovery Workshop, consultant or advisory role
Justin C. Deskovich, DPT, MPT, OCS, SCS, DAC, CSCS, COMT, FAAOMPT, FMS Cert.: Nemacolin Woodlands Resort, consultant
Jeannette Q. Lee, PT, PhD: Medcom, consultant or advisory role; UCSF Helen Diller Family Comprehensive Cancer Center, research funding
Alaina Newell, PT, DPT, WCS, CLT-LANA: American Physical Therapy Association section of Women's Health, research funding

Contents

Foreword

How crazy does it sound to be told to exercise when you are exhausted from the effects of chemotherapy? "I'm too tired to exercise." I used to say this over and over. It just didn't make sense to me. "Try it, Liz. You will feel so much better," my oncology nurse would say. Other nurses didn't know much about the relationship between fatigue and exercise and did not recommend anything to me.

When I was in the hospital, I had to walk around the unit at least twice before they would discharge me. Once I got home, I was still pretty sick. I started by walking around my dining room table. A few laps around the dining table may seem silly, but it was as much as I could tolerate and served as a good start. As I got some of my strength back, I walked around the perimeter of our house. I then graduated to walking outside through various culs-de-sac in my neighborhood. At one point I was up to walking five miles per day! I did not walk like that when I was healthy, before this cancer invaded my body.

For me, I began to notice a difference in the way I felt on days that I did not walk. Fighting the weather and having snow in the spring played serious havoc with my exercise schedule, and I would be disappointed when I could not go outdoors for my walk. I did get a chance to get out and about when we had warm, sunny weather in February and March of this past year. I would wear my Fitbit and sing along to the music on my phone. I got to know the neighbors better and even learned their dogs' names!

We turned these walks into a family affair. My husband would come along, my son and I would go out, each of my daughters walked with me separately, and one walk included everyone in the family—even the dog! It really was wonderful, and I am looking forward to warm weather when we can start going out again. When I walk with just one child, I have his or her complete, undivided attention. We have really good and meaningful talks during those times.

By exercising, not only do I feel better, but it feels like I can sleep more soundly. It even helps me deal with the pain related to the cancer. The one challenge that remains is my cognitive function. Writing my own book, *I'm Not That Person Anymore: A Nurse's Journey Living With Metastatic Breast Cancer*, has helped me focus my mind and inspired me to keep moving and exercising. I'm hopeful that exercise enhances my circulation, gets some more blood pumping into my brain, and helps me to remember things.

This book is incredibly important for oncology nurses, physical and occupational therapists, and oncology team members. These chapters explain the important connections between exercise and fatigue, pain, sleep, and cognitive function and how all nurses can recommend physical activity to their patients and cancer survivors. Nurses in the emergency department, intensive care unit, and medical-surgical units all take care of patients with cancer. They can all make recommendations for physical activity and exercise that are safe, tolerable, and doable. You can apply the information in this book in your practice and incorporate ideas and evidence to show cancer survivors how much better they can feel when participating in physical activity and exercise.

For cancer survivors who cannot walk, this book offers alternative options for physical activity, such as activities performed lying down, seated, and standing. For me, walking has been the best. Other cancer survivors may prefer to go to their local YMCA or community center. I have some friends who all get together and go to the YMCA for a swim class. They love it and feel like they are getting the type of exercise that is more applicable to them.

I am honored to read this book and write this foreword. I believe all nurses will find that they can better support cancer survivors after reading the evidence and processes presented in these chapters.

Elizabeth Wertz Evans, PhD, RN, MPM, CPHQ, CPHIMS, FHIMSS, FACMPE

Editors' note: Dr. Evans passed away prior to the publication of this book. Her enthusiasm and support for nursing, patient safety, and cancer care will be greatly missed.

Preface

Nearly 14.5 million children and adults with a history of cancer were alive on January 2014 in the United States alone (American Cancer Society [ACS], 2014). This number is expected to increase to an estimated 19 million cancer survivors by January 2024 (ACS, 2014). Ways to increase life expectancy and improve cancer treatment–related symptoms among cancer survivors include adopting healthy lifestyle patterns such as participating in a regular program of physical activity and exercise.

In 1989, two oncology nurses, Dr. Mary MacVicar and Dr. Maryl Winningham, published the seminal research on the effects of aerobic exercise on nausea (Winningham & MacVicar, 1988), functional capacity (MacVicar, Winningham, & Nickel, 1989), and body composition (Winningham, MacVicar, Bondoc, Anderson, & Minton, 1989) in breast cancer survivors. Not only did aerobic exercise reduce nausea and improve functional capacity and lean muscle mass in the breast cancer survivors, but it also was deemed safe for breast cancer survivors to perform. Over 25 years later, the foundation laid by these oncology nurses continues in the specialized field of exercise–oncology research.

Today, established and emerging evidence has solidified the relationship between physical activity and exercise and cancer survivorship. Evidence supports the ability of physical activity and exercise to ameliorate the effects of cancer-related treatments to improve sleep and cognitive function and reduce pain and fatigue. Physical activity is an important palliative care modality during cancer rehabilitation and end-of-life care.

Oncology nurses are well positioned to recommend physical activity to patients and their families. Nurses are trusted and are vested in patients' care. People living with cancer want to learn about physical activity—when and how to participate and how physical activity can keep them healthy—and they want to learn about it from their oncology nurse and physician (Bernardo, Abt, Ren, & Bender, 2010).

This book guides oncology nurses in the process of promoting physical activity for cancer survivors. This process includes assessing for physical and psychosocial readiness to participate in physical activity, recommending physical activity based on principles of exercise science, and evaluating outcomes associated with physical activity in cancer survivors. Best practices related to types of physical activities that are most appropriate for cancer survivors are discussed and are aligned with the *Statement on the Scope and Standards of Oncology Nursing Practice: Generalist and Advanced Practice* (Brant & Wickham, 2013). Basic principles of physical activity planning are presented in addition to ways to assess physical and psychosocial readiness to participate in physical activity and exercise. Also included in this book is the application of national guidelines and evidence to improve symptom-specific (cognitive functioning, pain, sleep, fatigue) and cancer-specific (lymphedema, cachexia, bone loss, metastasis) aspects of the cancer trajectory.

Collaboration and consultation with an interprofessional healthcare team, such as physical and occupational therapists, pharmacists, and exercise scientists, is emphasized. Survivor health conditions that require referral to specialty services such as physical therapy, rehabilitative medicine, and nutrition services are included. Oncology nurses can compare and contrast this book's evidence against their oncology center's protocols to strengthen and enhance their nursing practice.

Patients deserve the opportunity to receive current and credible guidance to incorporate physical activity into their lives throughout the cancer experience. Oncology nurses and team members knowledgeable about appropriate physical activities can improve cancer survivors' quality of life and health outcomes.

References

American Cancer Society. (2014). *Cancer treatment and survivorship facts and figures 2014–2015.* Retrieved from http://www.cancer.org/acs/groups/content/@research/documents/document/acspc-042801.pdf

Bernardo, L.M., Abt, K., Ren, D., & Bender, C. (2010). Self-reported exercise during breast cancer treatment: Results of a national survey. *Cancer Nursing, 33,* 304–309. doi:10.1097/NCC.0b013e3181cdce2c

Brant, J., & Wickham, R. (Eds.). (2013). *Statement on the scope and standards of oncology nursing practice: Generalist and advanced practice.* Pittsburgh, PA: Oncology Nursing Society.

MacVicar, M.G., Winningham, M.L., & Nickel, J.L. (1989). Effects of aerobic interval training on cancer patients functional capacity. *Nursing Research, 38,* 348–351. doi:10.1097/00006199-198911000-00007

Winningham, M.L., & MacVicar, M.G. (1988). The effect of aerobic exercise on patient reports of nausea. *Oncology Nursing Forum, 15,* 447–450.

Winningham, M.L., MacVicar, M.G., Bondoc, M., Anderson, J.I., & Minton, J.P. (1989). Effect of aerobic exercise on body weight and composition in patients with breast cancer on adjuvant chemotherapy. *Oncology Nursing Forum, 16,* 683–689.

Acknowledgments

Special thanks to Fran Higgins, MA, ADWR, of the College of Allied Health Professions, University of Nebraska Medical Center, and Morris "Rick" Brato of the University of Central Florida for their photo work in capturing active lifestyles.

CHAPTER **1**

Overview

Kathryn E. Tasillo, PT, DPT

Introduction

Whether it's walking to the mailbox, planting a garden, or cleaning the house, physical activity is a part of everyone's life. However, most Americans, including cancer survivors, do not regularly engage in daily physical activity. According to data from the National Health Interview Survey, 47% of adults did not meet the federal guidelines for participation in aerobic and muscle-strengthening activities (Blackwell, Lucas, & Clarke, 2014). A study of cancer survivors showed that only 47% of cancer survivors met the 2009 federal recommendations for weekly physical activity (Nayak, Holmes, Nguyen, & Elting, 2014).

Regular physical activity promotes health and prevents disease. For cancer survivors, physical activity is a means to not only promote health but also to ameliorate side effects (e.g., fatigue, pain) and promote cognitive functioning, sleep, and blood count recovery. Regular exercise improves balance, decreases risk of falls, improves circulation to the legs, helps survivors to maintain independence, decreases nausea, prevents muscle wasting, and improves self-esteem (American Cancer Society, 2014). Furthermore, physical activity is associated with increased rates of cancer survivorship. Chapter 2 provides current evidence demonstrating the association between exercise and physical activity and cancer survivorship.

Patients with cancer often ask their oncology nurses about physical activity during and after cancer treatment. Should they rest or be physically active? What are the appropriate physical activities for this population? Is there a certain "dose" of physical activity that is right for cancer survivors? The purpose of this chapter is to introduce the concept of physical activity and review the roles of healthcare and fitness professionals who promote physical activity. Different ways to open the discussion with cancer survivors about the value of physical activity are also presented. This chapter's content is supported by elements of the Oncology Nursing Society's (ONS's) *Statement on the Scope and Standards of Oncology Nursing Practice: Generalist and Advanced Practice* (Brant & Wickham, 2013) (see Figure 1-1).

Standard I. Assessment
• Communicate assessment data in a timely manner with appropriate providers and members of the interdisciplinary cancer care team.

Standard II. Diagnosis
• Develop and/or validate nursing diagnoses with the patient, family, and appropriate providers, including the interdisciplinary cancer care team when possible.

Standard III. Outcome Identification
• Develop expected outcomes collaboratively with the patient, family, interdisciplinary cancer care team, and other providers when possible.
• Ensure that expected outcomes are realistic in relation to the patient's present and potential capabilities.
• Design expected outcomes to maximize the patient's functional abilities.

Standard IV. Planning
• Incorporate appropriate preventive, therapeutic, rehabilitative, and palliative nursing actions into each phase of the plan of care along the cancer trajectory.
• Develop the plan of care in collaboration with the patient, family, interdisciplinary cancer care team, and other healthcare professionals when possible.
• Coordinate appropriate resources and consultative services to provide continuity of care and appropriate follow-up in the plan of care.
• Communicate the plan of care to other healthcare professionals and the interdisciplinary cancer care team.

Standard V. Implementation
• Identify community resources and support systems needed to implement the plan of care.

Standard VI. Evaluation
• Ensure that the patient, family, and members of the interdisciplinary cancer care team participate collaboratively in the evaluation process when possible.
• Communicate the patient's response with the interdisciplinary cancer care team and other agencies involved in the healthcare continuum.

Figure 1-1. Standards Applicable to Patient Care

Note. From *Statement on the Scope and Standards of Oncology Nursing Practice: Generalist and Advanced Practice,* by J.M. Brant and R. Wickham (Eds.), 2013, Pittsburgh, PA: Oncology Nursing Society. Copyright 2013 by Oncology Nursing Society. Adapted with permission.

Physical Activity and Living With Cancer

Physical activity is an umbrella term that describes bodily movement to accomplish activities of daily living. Table 1-1 shows types of physical activities and examples of activities for each category.

Table 1-1. Categories and Examples of Physical Activities

Activity Type	Category	Examples
Activities of daily living and instrumental activities of daily living	Occupational	Bathing Dressing Grooming
	Household	Vacuuming Dusting Washing dishes Doing laundry
Leisure activities	Transportation	Walking Running Bicycling
	Competitive sports*	Racquet sports Contact sports
	Recreational	Gardening Water activities Mall walking
	Exercise	Cardiovascular Strength and conditioning Flexibility (e.g., yoga, tai chi)

*Use caution with these sports, and consult with a physician to determine if appropriate to participate in regard to blood values, presence of an ostomy or wound, postsurgery, bone metastases, and other health conditions.

Current evidence and best practices support the value and importance of incorporating physical activity in the lifestyle of cancer survivors. For some cancer survivors, physical activity is familiar and a source of normalcy and comfort. For others, being physically active is new. Over time, cancer survivors should be educated on how to slowly incorporate physical activity into their lifestyle to improve their activity level and quality of life (American Cancer Society, 2014).

Most cancer survivors would like to learn about physical activity and different ways to be physically active. These individuals typically request information about physical activity early in their treatment and at more than one appointment. Overwhelmingly, cancer survivors indicate that they prefer to receive information from their oncology nurse (James-Martin, Koczwara, Smith, & Miller, 2014; Keogh, Patel, MacLeod, & Masters, 2014). It is crucial that oncology nurses, the oncology healthcare team, families, and organizations promote physical activity using the best evidence and practice guidelines. Chapter 3 discusses ways to promote physical activity in patients, families, and organizations.

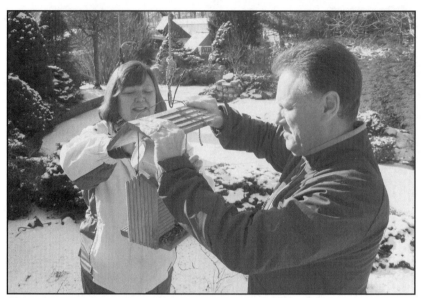

Physical activity is body movement that accomplishes activities of daily living. Feeding birds is an example of a recreational activity.

The Science of Physical Activity

The science of physical activity is grounded in *exercise science*. Exercise science is a specialty that studies human movement intended to maintain or improve physical fitness. This specialty includes exercise physiology, exercise psychology, cardiac rehabilitation, athletic training, and fitness for special populations. Exercise science principles are used to prescribe and recommend physical activities and physical activity programs for healthy populations as well as for those living with chronic diseases, such as cancer. Chapter 3 outlines these basic principles, and Chapters 4, 5, 6, and 7 synthesize these principles with current evidence to create and evaluate physical activity programs appropriate for cancer survivors.

Oncology nurses can guide cancer survivors to integrate physical activity as a lifestyle approach throughout cancer survivorship. Chapter 2 details the evidence relating to physical activity and cancer survivorship.

Oncology nurses can promote physical activity in cancer survivors by doing the following:
- Encouraging family and friends to be active with the cancer survivor
- Selecting physical activities that are enjoyable for the cancer survivor
- Promoting physical activities based on the cancer survivor's fatigue, cognitive functioning, pain, and sleep status. Chapters 8, 9, 10, and 11 provide current evidence and physical activity recommendations for these conditions.

- Selecting physical activities based on cancer-related considerations (e.g., lymphedema). Chapter 12 reviews current evidence for physical activity guidelines for lymphedema, cachexia, and bone loss. Chapter 13 offers current evidence for physical activity related to metastatic disease and end-of-life or palliative care.
- Selecting physical activities based on the cancer survivor's environment (e.g., hospital inpatient or outpatient setting, home, community, workplace) and stage of survivorship (see Table 1-2)

Table 1-2. Suggested Physical Activities During and After Cancer Treatment

Environment	Activities	Nursing Considerations
Inpatient and outpatient setting	In bed: • Breathing (in through nose, out through mouth) • Head rolls and head turns • Shoulder rolls and shrugs • Arm lifts • Fists open and close • Wrist circles • Ankle pumps and circles • Heel slides • Straight leg raises • Legs out and in (like a snow angel) Sitting on the edge of the bed or in a chair: • Breathing (in through nose, out through mouth) • Head rolls and head turns • Shoulder rolls and shrugs • Arm lifts • Punch (shoulder) forward • Punch (shoulder) across to opposite shoulder • Seated marching (bending and straightening the leg) • Heel/toe taps Standing with an assistive device or at a countertop: • Standing marches • Mini squats/chair squats • Swinging legs out to the side (hip abduction)	If inpatient, observe patients' mobility; discuss level of physical activity at home and compare to inpatient status. Obtain consult for physical therapist (PT) or occupational therapist (OT) in patients demonstrating diminished ability to safely ambulate, transfer, or perform activities of daily living independently or impaired sensation from chemotherapy-induced neuropathy. Follow PT or OT prescription for patients' therapy. Activities are completed gently at the pace and duration determined by the patient (low intensity). Use family members to enhance mobility if safe and appropriate.

(Continued on next page)

Table 1-2. Suggested Physical Activities During and After Cancer Treatment *(Continued)*

Environment	Activities	Nursing Considerations
Inpatient and outpatient setting *(cont.)*	• Lifting legs out back while keeping back straight (hip extension) • Heel/toe raises • Walking in the room or hallway (with or without assistance or assistive device) • Performing self-care as close to home level as possible	
Home setting	Moderate activities: • Walking • Cycling • Gardening • Dancing • Water aerobics • Golfing (without a cart) Vigorous activities: • Running • Fast walking • Heavy yard work • Swimming laps • Aerobics • Basketball	Help patients identify activities that are enjoyable, such as dancing, gardening, or mall walking. Encourage patients to find an exercise partner, keep a log or journal, set goals, and provide rewards for accomplishing goals and staying active; keep it fun!
Community setting	Yoga and tai chi classes	Yoga and tai chi help with stretching and balance, which can become affected by chemotherapy-induced neuropathy in the legs. The meditation component can be an additional benefit.

Provide patients with these suggestions regardless of activity/setting:
• Slowly increase the activity level with gentle warm-ups and cooldowns pre- and post-workout
• Stay hydrated; carry a water bottle during activities.
• Begin activities, such as walking or gardening, on flat surfaces.
• Pay attention to any numbness or decreased sensation in the feet; if present, use a recumbent cycle instead of a treadmill.
• Increase activity level according to activity level prior to the cancer diagnosis.
• Join an exercise group of cancer survivors.

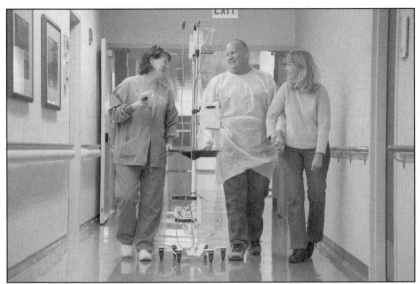

Being physically active while hospitalized is important to maintain muscle mass, strength, and aerobic capacity. Nurses can encourage patients to walk with family members during their stay.

A Team Approach to Physical Activity

Along the spectrum of cancer treatment and care, cancer survivors will likely work with various healthcare, fitness, and recreation professionals who can help them stay physically active.

During clinic visits and hospitalization periods, it is crucial for patients to remain active in accordance with their health status. Oncology nurses can be proactive when promoting appropriate physical activities for their patients by assuming responsibility for initiating and maintaining these activities in accordance with oncology nursing practice guidelines. When oncology nurses in hospital settings assume responsibility for their patients' physical activity and exercise, they are promoting their patients' health. As noted by Doherty-King and Bowers (2013), "Nurses who claimed responsibility for ambulation focused on patient independence and psychosocial well-being. This resulted in actions related to collaborating with physical therapy, determining the appropriateness of activity orders, diminishing the risk, and adjusting to resource availability" (p. 1240).

When living at home, survivors may engage in various physical activities (e.g., garden clubs, walking groups). Cancer survivors with functional mobility deficits can receive physical and occupational therapy in the home or in the outpatient clinic during ongoing cancer treatments. Table 1-3 outlines the

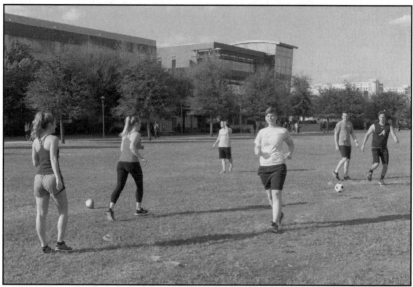

For cancer survivors, physical activity promotes health and is associated with increased rates of cancer survivorship. Soccer is a great example of a vigorous physical activity.

roles, responsibilities, and qualifications of healthcare and fitness professionals who may work with cancer survivors. Oncology nurses can consult with these professionals when recommending physical activity options for their patients.

Empowering Cancer Survivors to Be Physically Active

Cancer survivors must be educated on the benefits of physical activity and empowered to make physical activity a regular part of their daily lives, even when they are fatigued or in pain. Oncology nurses can empower cancer survivors by doing the following:

> "I had to learn how to listen to my body and nudge it toward recovery slowly, patiently, and intentionally. In developing goals, exercises, and the determination to be 'tall' again, I am forever in debt to the physical therapists in the hospital and to those who came to my home (after I was discharged) to encourage, support, and remind me that a 'new me' emerged."
>
> —Ron A.

- Eliciting the support of family and friends in making physical activity a priority
- Assessing individual activity preferences and abilities and matching these with physical activities that are best for each survivor

Table 1-3. Roles and Responsibilities of Health and Fitness Professionals

Professional	Role and Responsibilities	Education	Practice Setting	Other
Physical therapist	Expert in mobility to restore pain-free function and optimize movement; provides education on prevention and wellness (American Physical Therapy Association, 2015)	Doctorate in physical therapy	Inpatient Outpatient Home Rehab Nursing home	May require prescription May be fee for service or covered by insurance
Occupational therapist	Helps patients with daily tasks at home, work, and school to engage in all they want and need to do (American Occupational Therapy Association, 2015)	Master's or doctorate in occupational therapy	Inpatient Outpatient Home Rehab Nursing home	May require prescription May be fee for service or covered by insurance
Exercise physiologist	Measures baseline cardiopulmonary status or fitness ability and designs exercise programs based on individuals' abilities	Master's degree in exercise science	Inpatient Outpatient Exercise facility	Insurance Usually consulted by physician
Recreational therapist	Plans, directs, and coordinates recreation-based treatment programs, including arts and crafts, drama, music, dance, sports, games, and community reintegration field trips	Bachelor's degree	Community-based recreational facility or health center	Facility may be minimal charge or free; private pay or insurance may cover
Group fitness instructor	Designs fitness programs for groups of individuals	High school education; certification may be obtained	Exercise facility	Private pay
Personal trainer	Designs exercise programs based on individuals' abilities	High school education and certification	Home Exercise facility	Private pay

- Offering modifications to physical activities to promote adherence when in pain, fatigued, or sleep deprived or with poor cognitive functioning or psychosocial well-being
- Offering resources (e.g., support groups, local fitness clubs, social media, apps) for individuals in the hospital and at home to help promote physical activity
- Teaching cancer survivors how to listen to their bodies and teaching family and friends to help recognize signs of fatigue, pain, poor cognitive functioning, sleep deprivation, and psychosocial changes
- Encouraging cancer survivors to ask for physical activity recommendations from their oncology team
- Encouraging cancer survivors to request referrals to physical and occupational therapists if their strength, general mobility level, and ability to perform activities of daily living are declining
- Participating in a regular program of physical activity to promote personal and professional growth. Such programs are set up through local fitness centers, YMCAs, hospital-based wellness centers, and other venues.
- Appreciating the ongoing research related to physical activity and cancer survivorship. Chapter 14 highlights ongoing clinical trials that are generating new evidence related to the value of physical activity and exercise in cancer survivors. Opportunities for professional involvement in generating and disseminating evidence are presented.
- Obtaining exercise programming certification to better serve cancer survivors. Chapter 15 includes information on how to become certified as a cancer exercise specialist and offers resources for oncology nurses and cancer survivors to learn more about physical activity and exercise.
- Applying existing resources for principles of physical activity and exercise science to oncology nursing practice. Chapter 15 lists professional and lay organizations that promote knowledge, skills, and abilities related to exercise science. Applicable resources include the following:
  - ONS's Putting Evidence Into Practice resources: www.ons.org/practice -resources/pep
  - ONS's Get Up, Get Moving campaign: www.ons.org/practice-resources/ get-up-get-moving
  - National Comprehensive Cancer Network® Clinical Practice Guidelines in Oncology (NCCN Guidelines®): www.nccn.org
  - American College of Sports Medicine exercise guidelines for cancer survivors: www.acsm.org/public-information/acsm-journals/guidelines

Application to Oncology Nursing Practice

1. Use this list of activities to assess the current status of physical activity recommendations in your practice and identify opportunities for practice improvement. If cancer survivors are unable to safely complete some of

the supine or sitting activities listed in Table 1-2, physical or occupational therapists should be consulted as to whether inpatient or outpatient therapy is appropriate to assist patients in returning to their baseline functional level.

2. Collaborate with your oncology center's physical and occupational therapists about activities that cancer survivors can safely perform while at home, at the oncology center, or while hospitalized. Physical therapists can create a discharge plan of recommended safe activities for cancer survivors. If physical or occupational therapists are not available in your facility, speak to the attending oncologist about a referral for outpatient clinic services.

3. Talk with your oncology team about how and when they discuss physical activity with cancer survivors during assessment. If physical activity is not routinely discussed with survivors, ask why this assessment is not conducted. Use this book to learn how to integrate the discussion, creation, and evaluation of physical activity in cancer survivors.

4. Refer to the resources in Chapter 15. Visit websites of organizations that are of interest to you. Learn more about physical activity programs and exercise science. Consider the qualifications for becoming a certified cancer exercise specialist. Learn more about the roles of physical and occupational therapists, as well as exercise physiologists, so that you can understand the assistance they provide to cancer survivors.

Summary

Physical activity looks different for everybody and every *body*. Cancer also looks different for every person and takes its toll on each individual's body differently. Physical activity should be viewed as a necessary component of the cancer treatment plan of care. The benefits of physical activity outweigh the risks during and after cancer treatment. The key is finding activities that are fun, enjoyable, and doable at home, as well as activities that promote strength and conditioning in the hospital. These routines will become lasting ones that improve overall well-being, quality of life, and survivorship.

References

American Cancer Society. (2014). Physical activity and the cancer patient. Retrieved from http://www.cancer.org/treatment/survivorshipduringandaftertreatment/stayingactive/physical-activity-and-the-cancer-patient

American Occupational Therapy Association. (2015). About occupational therapy. Retrieved from http://www.aota.org

American Physical Therapy Association. (2015). The physical therapist scope of practice. Retrieved from http://www.apta.org/ScopeofPractice

Blackwell, D.L., Lucas, J.W., & Clarke, T.C. (2014). Summary health statistics for U.S. adults: National Health Interview Survey, 2012. National Center for Health Statistics. *Vital and Health Statistics, 10*(260), 1–161. Retrieved from http://www.cdc.gov/nchs/data/series/sr_10/sr10_260.pdf

Brant, J.M., & Wickham, R. (Eds.). (2013). *Statement on the scope and standards of oncology nursing practice: Generalist and advanced practice.* Pittsburgh, PA: Oncology Nursing Society.

Doherty-King, B., & Bowers, B.J. (2013). Attributing the responsibility for ambulating patients: A qualitative study. *International Journal of Nursing Studies, 50*, 1240–1246. doi:10.1016/j.ijnurstu.2013.02.007

James-Martin, G., Koczwara, B., Smith, E.L., & Miller, M.D. (2014). Information needs of cancer patients and survivors regarding diet, exercise, and weight management: A qualitative study. *European Journal of Cancer Care, 23*, 340–348. doi:10.1111/ecc.12159

Keogh, J.W.L., Patel, A., MacLeod, R.D., & Masters, J. (2014). Perceived barriers and facilitators to physical activity in men with prostate cancer: Possible influence of androgen deprivation therapy. *European Journal of Cancer Care, 23*, 263–273. doi:10.1111/ecc.12141

Nayak, P., Holmes, H.M., Nguyen, H.T., & Elting, L.S. (2014). Self-reported physical activity among middle-aged cancer survivors in the United States: Behavioral Risk Factor Surveillance System Survey, 2009. *Preventing Chronic Disease, 11*, E156. doi:10.5888/pcd11.140067

CHAPTER 2

Physical Activity and Cancer Survival

Kerry S. Courneya, PhD, Andria R. Morielli, MSc, and Linda Trinh, PhD

Introduction

Perhaps the most compelling question for many cancer survivors is whether physical activity and exercise can lower their risk of cancer recurrence and improve survival rates (Courneya, Rogers, Campbell, Vallance, & Friedenreich, 2015). Physical activity may lower the risk of recurrence, cancer-specific mortality, and all-cause mortality in breast, colorectal, and prostate cancer survivors. Evidence supports that adopting even a modest physical activity program may enhance longevity following cancer treatment.

Oncology nurses are well positioned to guide cancer survivors in their selection of physical activities. Oncology nurses' understanding of anatomy, physiology, behavior change, and oncology treatment blends well with the science of physical activity. Combining nursing science and physical activity science provides oncology nurses with the foundation to recommend appropriate physical activities for cancer survivors.

This chapter reviews possible mechanisms for how physical activity may help improve cancer outcomes. The emerging epidemiologic evidence examining the association between exercise and cancer outcomes in breast, colorectal, prostate, and other cancer survivor groups is also discussed. This chapter's content is supported in the Oncology Nursing Society's *Statement on the Scope and Standards of Oncology Nursing Practice: Generalist and Advanced Practice* (Brant & Wickham, 2013) (see Figure 2-1).

Standard IX. Evidence-Based Practice and Research
- Regularly access nationally recognized clinical practice guidelines (e.g., Oncology Nursing Society's position statements and Putting Evidence Into Practice resources; American Society of Clinical Oncology and National Comprehensive Cancer Network clinical practice guidelines) to support evidence-based patient care and teaching.
- Base clinical decision making and delivery of individualized patient care on best current evidence, patient values and preferences, and resource availability.
- Facilitate integration of new evidence into standards of practice, development or modification of policies, practice guidelines, education, and clinical management strategies.

Standard X. Quality of Practice
- Participate in quality assessment and improvement activities related to personal position and practice setting such as the following:
  - Formulate recommendations based on identification of discrepancies between current and optimal practice and developing action plans that address options for improving nursing and interprofessional care.
  - Integrate evidence-based findings into clinical practice.
  - Develop policies, guidelines, protocols, and order sets that translate and assimilate national standards of care into individual practice settings.

Standard XI. Communication
- Assess the patient's readiness, willingness, and ability to communicate, potential barriers to effective communication, and patient preferences for communication method and adapt communication style and method based on patient preferences and needs.
- Use established communication strategies to address potential communication barriers related to language, culture, sensory or cognitive challenges, or psychosocial disorders to enhance the patient's and family's understanding of the care plan.

Standard XII. Leadership
- Anticipate oncology and healthcare trends with changes such as innovative practice settings and models of care delivery, increased focus on older adult patients and cancer survivors, and technological advances that affect care.

Figure 2-1. Standards Applicable to Research on Cancer Survival

Note. From *Statement on the Scope and Standards of Oncology Nursing Practice: Generalist and Advanced Practice,* by J.M. Brant and R. Wickham (Eds.), 2013, Pittsburgh, PA: Oncology Nursing Society. Copyright 2013 by Oncology Nursing Society. Adapted with permission.

How Physical Activity May Improve Cancer Outcomes

The association between physical activity and cancer outcomes is independent from body mass index or obesity, suggesting that cancer survivors may benefit from physical activity even if they do not lose weight.

Possible biological factors and other mechanisms that may explain the associations between physical activity and cancer survival include the following (Winzer, Whiteman, Reeves, & Pratz, 2011):
- Metabolic hormones and growth factors
- Immune system

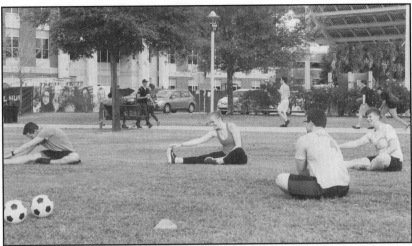

Evidence supports exercise and physical activity to promote cancer survivorship.

- Regulation of energy balance and fat distribution
- Antioxidant defense and DNA repair
- Insulin and insulin-like growth factors, natural killer cell cytotoxicity, and C-reactive protein
- Alterations in sex steroid hormones
- Decreased gastrointestinal transit time
- Improved pulmonary ventilation and perfusion
    Indirect ways in which physical activity may improve cancer outcomes include the following:
- Increased treatment options
- Improved treatment completion rates
- Better treatment response
- Reduced death rates from non–cancer-related causes

Physical Activity and Energy Expenditure

Research studies with cancer survivors demonstrate that even low-MET activities affect cancer survival rates.

    Physical activity expends energy; this energy is measured as metabolic equivalent of tasks (METs). One MET is the rate of energy expended while resting. METs associated with numerous physical activities are described in Chapter 4. Examples include the following:
- Light (< 3 METs) activities: strolling, slow walking
- Moderate (3–6 METs) activities: brisk walking, light bicycling
- Vigorous (> 6 METs) activities: jogging, jumping rope

Physical Activity and Breast Cancer Outcomes

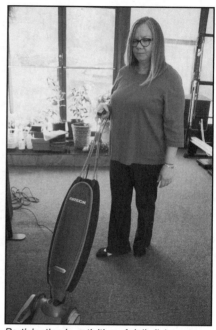

Participating in activities of daily living promotes cancer survivorship.

Most of the research on physical activity and cancer outcomes is focused on breast cancer. Two of the earliest epidemiologic studies on physical activity and breast cancer outcomes are particularly informative. For an average of eight years, Holmes, Chen, Feskanich, Kroenke, and Colditz (2005) followed 2,987 women from the Nurses' Health Study who were diagnosed with stages I–III breast cancer between 1984 and 1998. Physical activity was assessed by self-report every two years. After adjusting for other important factors, including an indicator of body fat called body mass index (BMI), analyses showed that women reporting 9–15 MET-hours per week of physical activity had a 50% lower risk of death from breast cancer compared to women reporting less than 3 MET-hours per week. Moreover, 10 years later, 92% of women who reported 9 or more MET-hours per week were still alive, compared to 86% of women reporting less than 3 MET-hours per week.

Holick et al. (2008) examined the association between postdiagnosis recreational physical activity and risk of breast cancer death in 4,482 breast cancer survivors enrolled in the Collaborative Women's Longevity Study. The women were aged 20–79 years and were an average of 5.6 years postdiagnosis when they participated in the study. Physical activity was assessed by self-report of six recreational activities over the first year, and the women were followed for up to six years. After adjusting for other important factors, including age, family history of breast cancer, disease stage, hormone therapy use, treatments, energy intake, and BMI, the women engaging in 2.8 or greater MET-hours per week of physical activity had a 40%–50% lower risk of breast cancer death and all-cause mortality. The association was similar regardless of age or stage of disease.

Two recent systematic reviews summarized the growing number of studies on exercise and breast cancer outcomes. Schmid and Leitzmann (2014) identified five studies examining postdiagnosis physical activity and breast cancer outcomes. High versus low postdiagnosis physical activity was associated with a decreased risk of total mortality (relative risk [RR] = 0.52; 95% confidence interval [CI] [0.42–0.64]) and breast cancer–specific mortality (RR = 0.72; 95% CI [0.60–0.85]). Each 5, 10, or 15 MET-hours-per-week increase in post-diagnosis physical activity was associated with a 13% (95% CI [6%–20%]), 24% (95% CI [11%–36%]), and 34% (95% CI [16%–38%]) decreased risk of total mortality, respectively, and a 6% (95% CI [3%–8%]), 11% (95% CI [6%–15%]), and 16% (95% CI [9%–22%]) reduction in risk of breast cancer–specific mortality, respectively. The association between postdiagnosis physical activity and total mortality did not differ according to BMI, menopausal status, or tumor estrogen receptor status.

In a more recent systematic review and meta-analysis, Lahart, Metsios, Nevill, and Carmichael (2015) examined the relationship between physical activity and all-cause mortality, breast cancer–specific mortality, and breast cancer recurrence. The review included 22 studies for a total of 123,574 participants; however, only nine studies examined postdiagnosis physical activity. For comparisons between the highest and lowest levels of self-reported postdiagnosis recreational physical activity, the hazard ratio (HR) was 0.52 (95% CI [0.43–0.64]) for all-cause mortality, 0.59 (95% CI [0.45–0.78]) for breast cancer–related mortality, and 0.79 (95% CI [0.63–0.98]) for breast cancer events.

Although the data on exercise and breast cancer outcomes are promising, studies have been limited by self-reported measures and secondary analyses of studies that were not originally designed to answer this question.

Oncology Nurse Recommendations for Physical Activity in Breast Cancer Survivors

Based on this body of evidence, oncology nurses can safely recommend physical activity for breast cancer survivors.
- Recommend physical activities that are in the moderate (3–6 METs) range of energy expenditure for all breast cancer survivors.
- Recommend physical activities that are in the vigorous (> 6 METs) range of energy expenditure for breast cancer survivors who enjoy this level of physical activity.

Physical Activity and Colorectal Cancer Outcomes

A growing number of studies have examined the link between physical activity and colorectal cancer outcomes, and the findings are very promising. Meyerhardt, Heseltine, et al. (2006) reported results of a prospective study of more than 800 colorectal cancer survivors with stage III disease who had participated in a chemotherapy trial. Physical activity was self-reported six months after completion of chemotherapy, and participants were followed for about 3.8 years.

Physical activity categories were predefined as the following: 3 or less, 3–8.9, 9–17.9, 18–26.9, and 27 or greater MET-hours per week. Analyses adjusted for BMI and other important factors indicated that higher levels of physical activity were associated with longer disease-free survival and overall survival. Specifically, after three years of follow-up, 85% of colorectal cancer survivors who exercised 18 or greater MET-hours per week were free of their disease, compared to 75% of those who exercised 18 or less MET-hours per week.

Meyerhardt, Giovannucci, et al. (2006) reported a prospective study of 573 women with stages I–III colorectal cancer. In this study, physical activity was self-reported before and after diagnosis, and analyses were again adjusted for important factors. Results showed that higher postdiagnosis physical activity was associated with a lower risk of death from colorectal cancer and death from all causes. Specifically, as compared with women exercising 3 or less MET-hours per week, the risk of death from colorectal cancer was 8% lower for women reporting 3–8.9 MET-hours per week, 43% lower for women reporting 9–17.9 MET-hours per week, and 61% lower for women reporting 18 or greater MET-hours per week. The risk of death from all causes was similarly reduced with increasing physical activity levels. Furthermore, women who increased their physical activity after diagnosis from their prediagnosis level had improved cancer outcomes compared to women who did not change their physical activity. Women who decreased their physical activity had poorer outcomes.

Finally, Meyerhardt et al. (2009) reported on 668 men diagnosed with stages I–III colorectal cancer as part of the Health Professionals Follow-Up Study. The results indicated that men who reported engaging in more than 27 MET-hours per week of physical activity had a 53% lower risk of colorectal cancer–specific mortality than men who reported engaging in less than 27 MET-hours per week of physical activity. Similarly, the risk for overall mortality was 41% lower. Moreover, the proportion of men alive at five years postdiagnosis was 85.2% for men who engaged in 3 or less MET-hours per week, compared to 87.4% of men engaging in 3–27 MET-hours per week and 92.1% for men engaging in more than 27 MET-hours per week. Finally, the 10-year survival rates for higher levels of physical activity were 79.4%, 81.2%, and 88.3%, respectively. These associations remained largely unchanged regardless of age, disease stage, BMI, time of diagnosis, tumor location, and prediagnosis physical activity level.

Two meta-analyses published in 2013 (Des Guetz et al., 2013; Je, Jeon, Giovannucci, & Meyerhardt, 2013) reviewed the same seven prospective colorectal cancer cohort studies. Six of the reviewed studies assessed the relationship between postdiagnosis physical activity level and colorectal cancer–specific mortality and all-cause mortality in 6,348 colorectal cancer survivors. Je et al. (2013) conducted a separate meta-analysis for (a) exercisers versus nonexercisers, (b) colorectal cancer survivors with moderate versus low physical activity levels, and (c) colorectal cancer survivors with high versus low physical activity levels. Overall, the results of the meta-analysis showed that participation in any physical activity postdiagnosis reduced the risk of colorectal cancer–specific mortality and all-cause mortality. Furthermore, participation in higher levels of postdiagnosis physical activity was associated with a greater reduction in risk for both colorectal cancer–specific mortality and all-cause mortality.

Oncology Nurse Recommendations for Physical Activity in Colorectal Cancer Survivors

Based on this body of evidence, oncology nurses can safely recommend physical activity for colorectal cancer survivors.
- Recommend physical activities that are in the moderate (3–6 METs) range of energy expenditure for all colorectal cancer survivors.
- Recommend physical activities that are in the vigorous (> 6 METs) range of energy expenditure for colorectal cancer survivors who enjoy this level of physical activity.

Physical Activity and Prostate Cancer Outcomes

A small number of studies have examined the association between exercise and prostate cancer outcomes, and the results have been promising. For example, a study by Kenfield, Stampfer, Giovannucci, and Chan (2011) examined the association between postdiagnosis physical activity and prostate cancer outcomes. Based on the Health Professionals Follow-Up Study of 51,529 male health professionals in the United States, 2,705 men diagnosed with nonmetastatic prostate cancer between 1990 and 2008 were included in the analysis. The results indicated that men who engaged in 9 or greater MET-hours per week versus those with less physical activity had a 35% lower risk of death from prostate cancer and a 33% lower risk of death from all causes. Both nonvigorous (defined as < 6 METs) and vigorous (defined as ≥ 6 METs) physical activity levels were associated with a reduced risk of all-cause mortality; however, only vigorous physical activity was associated with a reduced risk of death from prostate cancer. Specifically, men who performed greater than three hours per week of vigorous physical activity compared to those who exercised for less than one hour per week at the same intensity had a 61% lower risk of prostate cancer–related death. Overall, this study suggests that moderate to vigorous physical activity may improve overall survival rates in prostate cancer.

Oncology Nurse Recommendations for Physical Activity in Prostate Cancer Survivors

Based on this body of evidence, oncology nurses can safely recommend physical activity for prostate cancer survivors.

- Recommend physical activities that are in the vigorous (> 6 METs) range of energy expenditure.
- Recommend physical activities that are in the light (< 3 METs) to moderate (3–6 METs) range of energy expenditure as a means to engage survivors in being physically active and with the intention of raising the level of activity intensity over time.

Physical Activity and Cancer Outcomes in Other Cancer Survivor Groups

Ovarian Cancer

A study by Moorman, Jones, Akushevich, and Schildkraut (2011) examined the association between prediagnosis physical activity and ovarian cancer survival. The analysis included 638 ovarian cancer survivors recruited from 1999 to 2008 in North Carolina. The results showed no association between prediagnosis physical activity and overall ovarian cancer survival. However, a suggestion of improved survival was noted for women in the healthy BMI range who reported physical activity greater than two hours per week compared to women reporting one hour per week.

Hematologic Cancer

Two recent randomized controlled trials have reported exploratory follow-up of cancer outcomes in hematologic cancer survivors. Courneya, Friedenreich, et al. (2015) reported an exploratory follow-up of progression-free survival (PFS) from the Healthy Exercise for Lymphoma Patients (HELP) trial. Researchers conducting the HELP trial randomized 122 patients with lymphoma between 2005 and 2008 to either a control group (n = 62) or 12 weeks of supervised aerobic exercise (n = 60). The researchers abstracted PFS events from medical records in 2013. After a median follow-up of 61 months, the adjusted five-year PFS was 64.8% for the exercise group compared with 65.0% for the control group (HR = 1.01; 95% CI [0.51–2.01]). In a post hoc analysis combining the three groups that received supervised exercise, the adjusted five-year PFS for the supervised exercise groups was 68.5%, compared to 59.0% for the group that received no supervised exercise (HR = 0.70; 95% CI [0.35–1.39]). This exploratory follow-up of the HELP trial suggested that supervised aerobic exercise may be associated with improved PFS in patients with lymphoma; however, larger trials designed to answer this question are needed.

Wiskemann et al. (2015) reported an exploratory follow-up of 103 allogeneic stem cell transplant recipients who had taken part in a randomized controlled exercise trial. Patients in the exercise group trained prior to hospital admission, during inpatient treatment, and for six to eight weeks following discharge. The exercise program consisted of a combination of endurance training and resistance training. Survival outcomes included nonrelapse mortality (NRM) and total mortality (TM) for events that either occurred only after discharge or all events that occurred in the two-year observational period following transplantation (including the hospitalization period). NRM for events that occurred after discharge was 4% in the exercise group and 13.5% in the control group (RR = 0.30; p = 0.086); NRM for all events was 26% in the exercise group and 36.5% in the control group (RR = 0.71; p = 0.29). Furthermore, TM for events after discharge was 12% in the exercise group and 28.3% in the control group (RR = 0.42; p = 0.030); TM for all events was 34% in the exercise group and 50.9% in the control group (RR = 0.67; p = 0.11). The data from this follow-up study suggest that exercise may be associated with improved survival in patients undergoing allogenic stem cell transplantation. However, larger trials focused on survival rates are needed.

Oncology Nurse Recommendations for Physical Activity in Other Cancer Survivors

Based on these few studies, oncology nurses can recommend daily physical activity to all cancer survivors to maintain overall health and well-being.

Application to Oncology Nursing Practice

1. Discuss one of the research studies with your oncology team. Compare and contrast the study sample and physical activities with your oncology center's population and recommended activities.
2. Review your oncology center's recommended physical activities for cancer survivors based on type of cancer (e.g., breast, colorectal, prostate). Decide if activities can be added or removed from these lists.
3. Explore how your oncology center can educate cancer survivors on how physical activity can improve cancer survival. Consider resources such as education materials, hospital television station programming, and social media outlets.

Summary

Research on physical activity and cancer survival has increased dramatically in the last decade and is producing exciting results. Longer survival and better-tolerated treatments have created the opportunity for cancer survivors to help themselves after their diagnosis. In addition to improvements in physical functioning, fatigue, and quality of life, a growing number of studies suggest that physical activity may lower the risk of recurrence, cancer-specific mortality, and all-cause mortality in breast, colorectal, and prostate cancer survivors. To date, however, no large-scale phase III randomized controlled trials have demonstrated that adopting a physical activity program after a cancer diagnosis can alter the course of the disease or extend overall survival. Nevertheless, the preliminary findings are positive, and phase III exercise trials with cancer outcomes are underway (see Chapter 14).

Oncology nurses can apply these findings in their practice with cancer survivors. Recommending moderate and vigorous physical activities that are appealing and practical will help cancer survivors maintain a level of activity that is best for their health.

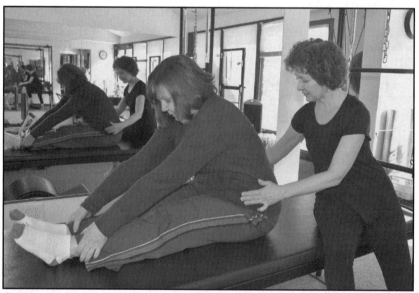

Stretching is a low metabolic equivalent activity that is important for warm-ups and cooldowns.

References

Brant, J.M., & Wickham, R. (Eds.). (2013). *Statement on the scope and standards of oncology nursing practice: Generalist and advanced practice.* Pittsburgh, PA: Oncology Nursing Society.

Courneya, K.S., Friedenreich, C.M., Franco-Villalobos, C., Crawford, J.J., Chua, N., Basi, S., ... Reiman, T. (2015). Effects of supervised exercise on progression-free survival in lymphoma patients: An exploratory follow-up of the HELP Trial. *Cancer Causes and Control, 26,* 269–276. doi:10.1007/s10552-014-0508-x

Courneya, K.S., Rogers, L.Q., Campbell, K.L., Vallance, J.K., & Friedenreich, C.M. (2015). Top 10 research questions related to physical activity and cancer survivorship. *Research Quarterly for Exercise and Sport, 86,* 107–116. doi:10.1080/02701367.2015.991265

Des Guetz, G., Uzzan, B., Bouillet, T., Nicolas, P., Chouahnia, K., Zelek, L., & Morere, J.F. (2013). Impact of physical activity on cancer-specific and overall survival of patients with colorectal cancer. *Gastroenterology Research and Practice, 2013,* Article ID 340851. doi:10.1155/2013/340851

Holick, C.N., Newcomb, P.A., Trentham-Dietz, A., Titus-Ernstoff, L., Bersch, A.J., Stampfer, M.J., ... Willett, W.C. (2008). Physical activity and survival after diagnosis of invasive breast cancer. *Cancer Epidemiology, Biomarkers and Prevention, 17,* 379–386. doi:10.1158/1055-9965.EPI-07-0771

Holmes, M.D., Chen, W.Y., Feskanich, D., Kroenke, C.H., & Colditz, G.A. (2005). Physical activity and survival after breast cancer diagnosis. *JAMA, 293,* 2479–2486. doi:10.1001/jama.293.20.2479

Je, Y., Jeon, J.Y., Giovannucci, E.L., & Meyerhardt, J.A. (2013). Association between physical activity and mortality in colorectal cancer: A meta-analysis of prospective cohort studies. *International Journal of Cancer, 133,* 1905–1913. doi:10.1002/ijc.28208

Kenfield, S.A., Stampfer, M.J., Giovannucci, E., & Chan, J.M. (2011). Physical activity and survival after prostate cancer diagnosis in the health professionals follow-up study. *Journal of Clinical Oncology, 29,* 726–732. doi:10.1200/JCO.2010.31.5226

Lahart, I.M., Metsios, G.S., Nevill, A.M., & Carmichael, A.R. (2015). Physical activity, risk of death and recurrence in breast cancer survivors: A systematic review and meta-analysis of epidemiological studies. *Acta Oncologica, 54,* 635–654. doi:10.3109/0284186X.2014.998275

Meyerhardt, J.A., Giovannucci, E.L., Holmes, M.D., Chan, A.T., Chan, J.A., Colditz, G.A., & Fuchs, C.S. (2006). Physical activity and survival after colorectal cancer diagnosis. *Journal of Clinical Oncology, 24,* 3527–3534. doi:10.1200/JCO.2006.06.0855

Meyerhardt, J.A., Giovannucci, E.L., Ogino, S., Kirkner, G.J., Chan, A.T., Willett, W., & Fuchs, C.S. (2009). Physical activity and male colorectal cancer survival. *Archives of Internal Medicine, 169,* 2102–2108. doi:10.1001/archinternmed.2009.412

Meyerhardt, J.A., Heseltine, D., Niedzwiecki, D., Hollis, D., Saltz, L.B., Mayer, R.J., ... Fuchs, C.S. (2006). Impact of physical activity on cancer recurrence and survival in patients with stage III colon cancer: Findings from CALGB 89803. *Journal of Clinical Oncology, 24,* 3535–3541. doi:10.1200/JCO.2006.06.0863

Moorman, P.G., Jones, L.W., Akushevich, L., & Schildkraut, J.M. (2011). Recreational physical activity and ovarian cancer risk and survival. *Annals of Epidemiology, 21,* 178–187. doi:10.1016/j.annepidem.2010.10.014

Schmid, D., & Leitzmann, M.F. (2014). Association between physical activity and mortality among breast cancer and colorectal cancer survivors: A systematic review and meta-analysis. *Annals of Oncology, 25,* 1293–1311. doi:10.1093/annonc/mdu012

Winzer, B.M., Whiteman, D.C., Reeves, M.M., & Pratz, J.D. (2011). Physical activity and cancer prevention: A systematic review of clinical trials. *Cancer Causes and Control, 22,* 811–826. doi:10.1007/s10552-011-9761-4

Wiskemann, J., Kleindienst, N., Kuehl, R., Dreger, P., Schwerdtfeger, R., & Bohus, M. (2015). Effects of physical exercise on survival after allogeneic stem cell transplantation. *International Journal of Cancer, 137,* 2749–2756. doi:10.1002/ijc.29633

CHAPTER **3**

Promoting Physical Activity for Cancer Survivors

Katrina Fetter, MSN, RN, OCN®

Introduction

Physical activity should be an important part of everybody's lives, and this is especially true for cancer survivors. RNs (particularly oncology nurses), hospital staff, and healthcare organizations should be knowledgeable about successful strategies to promote physical activity. Unfortunately, hospitalized patients and cancer survivors do not receive the benefit of this knowledge.

- About one-third of the average patient population receives physical activity recommendations from their healthcare provider (Centers for Disease Control and Prevention, 2012).
- Less than 10% of breast cancer survivors receive recommendations on physical activity from their healthcare provider (Fessele, Yendro, & Mallory, 2014).
- Cancer survivors are willing and feel able to participate in exercise (Blaney, Lowe-Strong, Rankin-Watt, Campbell, & Gracey, 2013).

This chapter explores the strategies that oncology nurses and their organizations can employ to promote physical activity in cancer survivors and their families. This chapter's content is supported in the Oncology Nursing Society's *Statement on the Scope and Standards of Oncology Nursing Practice: Generalist and Advanced Practice* (Brant & Wickham, 2013) (see Figure 3-1).

Standard I. Assessment
• Collect data from multiple sources, including the patient, the family, other care providers, and the community.

Standard II. Diagnosis
• Use evidence-based research to formulate the plan of care.

Standard III. Outcome Identification
• Ensure that expected outcomes are realistic in relation to the patient's present and potential capabilities.
• Design expected outcomes to maximize the patient's functional abilities.
• Formulate expected outcomes in congruence with other planned therapies and recognize how planned cancer therapies influence expected outcomes.
• Ensure that expected outcomes provide direction for continuity of care.
• Assign a realistic time period for expected outcomes for achievement or reevaluation and be aware of the timing of side effects and normal physiologic events associated with cancer treatment and align expected outcomes accordingly.

Standard IV. Planning
• Incorporate appropriate preventive, therapeutic, rehabilitative, and palliative nursing actions into each phase of the plan of care along the cancer trajectory.
• Ensure that the plan of care reflects sensitivity and respect for the patient's religious, spiritual, social, cultural, and ethnic practices.
• Include individualized physical, psychological, and social interventions in the plan of care that are
  – Supported by current evidence-based research and practice
  – Designed to achieve the stated outcomes
  – Prioritized according to the patient's needs and preferences
  – Supportive of diversity awareness
• Incorporate patient and family education and specific teaching plans into the plan of care, focusing on the 14 high-incidence problem areas.

Standard V. Implementation
• Ensure that interventions are implemented in a safe, culturally competent, appropriate, caring, and humanistic manner.
• Implement interventions with the concurrence and/or participation of the patient and family when possible.
• Use evidence-based research to guide implementation of interventions.
• Identify community resources and support systems needed to implement the plan of care.

Standard VI. Evaluation
• Ensure that the patient, family, and members of the interdisciplinary cancer care team participate collaboratively in the evaluation process when possible.

Figure 3-1. Standards Applicable to Promoting Physical Activity for Cancer Survivors

---

Note. From *Statement on the Scope and Standards of Oncology Nursing Practice: Generalist and Advanced Practice,* by J.M. Brant and R. Wickham (Eds.), 2013, Pittsburgh, PA: Oncology Nursing Society. Copyright 2013 by Oncology Nursing Society. Adapted with permission.

Overcoming Survivor- and Family-Related Barriers to Physical Activity

Cancer survivors, as well as those close to them, may struggle with meeting physical activity requirements for a variety of reasons. Survivors' families, friends, or significant others may exert a negative influence with their own personal beliefs, values, and preferences. Barriers to participating in physical activity include the following:
- Personal beliefs and attitudes toward physical activity and exercise
- Treatment-related issues
- Environmental barriers
- Lack of time
- Lack of social support
- Financial challenges
- Knowledge barriers

Table 3-1 provides examples of these barriers and outlines strategies that oncology nurses can use to overcome these barriers for cancer survivors and their families.

One of the most important ways to promote physical activity is by helping cancer survivors develop self-efficacy (Olson et al., 2014). Self-efficacy is an individual's belief in his or her capability to do something (Bandura, 1997). Without this belief or confidence, it is difficult for the individual to successfully participate in physical activities.

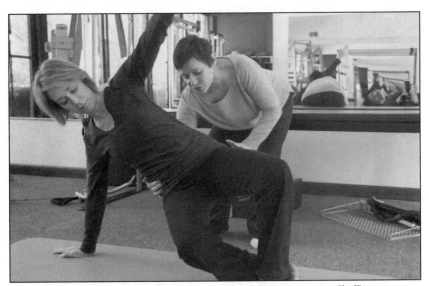

Reinforcing the benefits of exercise on physical health helps promote self-efficacy.

Table 3-1. Survivor-Related Barriers and Oncology Nursing Strategies for Promoting Physical Activity

Barrier	Examples	Suggested Nursing Strategies
Personal belief and attitude toward physical activity	Lack of interest in participating in physical activity	Educate and encourage the importance of activity while assessing motivation to change behavior.
	Preference for activities that do not involve physical activity	Inquire about enjoyable activities; suggest ways to incorporate physical activity into these enjoyable activities.
	The belief that the survivor is sick and needs to rest	Educate on the reasons why physical activity helps reduce fatigue (see Chapter 8) and improve survival (see Chapter 2).
	The idea that physical activity is not a priority, does not have benefits, and is therefore unnecessary	Educate about the proven positive effects of physical activity on cancer survivorship (see Chapter 2). Encourage cancer survivors who are physically active to meet with inactive cancer survivors. Direct individuals to support groups and cancer-specific activity programs (see Chapter 15).
	Lack of confidence in the ability to be physically active (usually due to a poor body image). For many individuals, additional fear and anxiety surround the concept of physical activity, especially in survivors with or at risk for lymphedema.	Reinforce that appropriate physical activity helps strengthen the body. This positive reinforcement helps survivors develop self-efficacy. Educate and demonstrate safe physical activities. Refer to physical therapy and occupational therapy for modifications for special considerations such as lymphedema (see Chapter 12).
Treatment	Fatigue, rated by 74% of survivors as the number-one barrier to physical activity. Often, survivors feel so tired that they do not want to participate in physical activity despite the fact that physical activity would actually help their fatigue.	Provide survivors with evidence reinforcing how physical activity helps with fatigue (see Chapter 8).

(Continued on next page)

Table 3-1. Survivor-Related Barriers and Oncology Nursing Strategies for Promoting Physical Activity *(Continued)*

Barrier	Examples	Suggested Nursing Strategies
Treatment *(cont.)*	Fear of worsening pain	Emphasize that pain is typically not worsened by appropriate physical activity and that pain can be addressed if it arises (see Chapter 10).
	Neuropathy	Reinforce with survivors that they can participate in physical activity even with neuropathy but may need to make adjustments for safety precautions. Refer to physical therapy or occupational therapy for activity modifications and assistive devices if needed.
	Depression	Discuss that many survivors with depression report improvement with physical activity.
	Cancer-specific barriers, for example, female survivors with breast cancer who avoid physical activity because their bras are uncomfortable and cause pain	Obtain properly fitting clothing, especially undergarments, to improve compliance with physical activity.
Environmental	Residing in neighborhoods that are unsafe or do not have sidewalks or safe places to engage in outdoor activities	Become familiar with local parks, recreation areas, and indoor venues (e.g., shopping malls) that are safe for physical activity (e.g., walking).
	Residing in rural areas that do not have fitness facilities or places to walk or do have facilities but require transportation to access them	Become familiar with transportation options for rural residents. Note if parks have physical activity stations where strength and flexibility activities can be added in addition to walking.
Time	Feeling of "being too busy." These individuals want physical activity opportunities easily available to them and at convenient times, which may not always be possible.	Offer ideas for physical activity that can be incorporated in their day (e.g., housework, walking up/down stairs). Direct them to resources for physical activities in their geographic area.

(Continued on next page)

Table 3-1. Survivor-Related Barriers and Oncology Nursing Strategies for Promoting Physical Activity (Continued)

Barrier	Examples	Suggested Nursing Strategies
Social support	Lack of social support, which leads to difficulties in successfully participating in a physical activity program	Encourage family, friends, and significant others to become involved in physical activity with survivors in order to increase success and compliance; this type of involvement gives survivors an outlet for getting help and support.
	Erroneous beliefs by social support systems that encourage survivors to rest and remain inactive	Use family, friends, and significant others for encouragement and role models for healthy behaviors. If survivors do not have a family member to get involved, find a fitness partner or cancer survivor and make an exercise agreement to improve activity adherence. Connect survivors with support groups either in person or online. Encourage survivors to reach out for support from family, friends, and significant others; include them in education and encourage their participation in survivor-related physical activity programs. Recruit survivors with similar physical activity interests to support other survivors in being physically active.
Financial	Inability to afford payment for fitness center membership or group	Locate free or reduced-cost or funded programs for their participation. Collaborate with the cancer center to develop physical activity programs for survivors.
Knowledge	Inability to access or find live or online programs to support physical activity	Collaborate with oncology team members, such as physical therapists, exercise scientists, and social services, to assist in finding appropriate no-cost or low-cost activity programs. Refer survivors to reputable online health and fitness sites.

(Continued on next page)

Table 3-1. Survivor-Related Barriers and Oncology Nursing Strategies for Promoting Physical Activity *(Continued)*

Barrier	Examples	Suggested Nursing Strategies
Knowledge *(cont.)*	Lack of discussion between survivors and oncology professionals regarding specific recommendations about physical activity	Assess, at each visit, survivors' physical activities. Discuss appropriate activities. Develop a plan for survivors to use (see Chapters 4 and 7).

Note. Based on information from Adams et al., 2014; Arroyave et al., 2008; Bandura, 1997; Barber, 2013; Forbes et al., 2014; Gho et al., 2014; Haas, 2011; James-Martin et al., 2014; Karvinen et al., 2012; Keogh et al., 2014; Olson et al., 2014; Sander et al., 2012; Schmitz et al., 2010; Spector et al., 2013.

Oncology nurses can familiarize themselves with the concept of self-efficacy and work to improve individuals' self-efficacy through verbal encouragement and activity programs that include a gradual increase of physical activity (Bakhshi, Sun, Murrells, & While, 2015; Haas, 2011). Considering the risks and benefits of physical activity and developing realistic goals with survivors also can help in establishing self-efficacy (Spector, Battaglini, & Groff, 2013). Chapter 5 discusses self-efficacy and motivational interviewing techniques oncology nurses can learn to promote positive behavior change in cancer survivors.

"My role as a patient forced me to find ways to help my medical team in understanding my recovery. I had to pay close attention to my body, the medications and their side effects, and to my own emotions in order to report back any changes and turbulences so my team would know how to react. Being physically active was a key ingredient in helping me move from 'patient' to 'survivor.'"

—Ron A.

One strategy to open the discussion on physical activity in cancer survivors is to ask individuals about their activity preferences. Many times, individuals may not realize their level of physical activity because they do not consider occupational activity (e.g., housework) a physical activity. Matching individuals' interests with appropriate activities will increase the chance of them becoming compliant and maintaining an interest in participating in physical activity (Forbes, Blanchard, Mummery, & Courneya, 2014; Spector et al., 2013). Dancing with family and friends, for example, may be much more enjoyable to an individual than walking; therefore, directing the individual and family on how to find and participate in dance classes or social dance venues will increase the likelihood of continued participation.

Individuals may also enjoy using computer programs, DVDs, or motivational tools (e.g., physical activity monitors, such as Fitbit® and Jawbone®) for physical activity that could help get them moving (Arroyave et al., 2008).

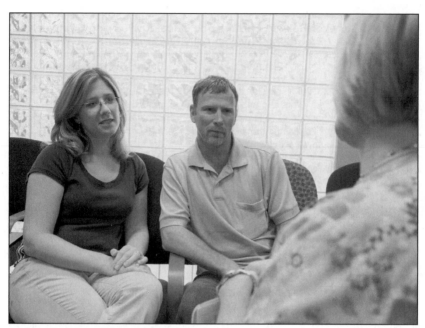

Asking about cancer survivors' preferences for physical activity will help oncology nurses to recommend appropriate activities.

Overcoming Oncology and Healthcare Professional Barriers to Promote Physical Activity and Exercise

Equally important to the efforts of improving adherence to physical activity is addressing the barriers faced by oncology nurses and healthcare professionals in recommending physical activity to cancer survivors (see Figure 3-2).

Table 3-2 outlines strategies that oncology nurses and healthcare professionals can employ to overcome these barriers. Becoming physically active needs to be an innate part of the healthcare professional's role (Bakhshi et al., 2015). In fact, as noted by Karvinen, McGourty, Parent, and Walker (2012), nurse-led physical activity interventions, such as walking programs, can be the most successful initiatives. They also serve as an effective way to engage cancer survivors and their families while also improving the oncology nurses' own perceptions of physical activity.

> One of the first strategies oncology nurses and other healthcare professionals can employ to recommend physical activity for cancer survivors is to evaluate their own participation in and attitudes toward physical activity. Healthcare professionals who embrace physical activity in their own lives serve as a model to their patients.

- Do not always exercise themselves and feel that they have little knowledge about physical activity
- Lack of awareness of the need to recommend physical activity and/or the benefits of physical activity
- No current organizational support or structure in place to find patients' current level of activity
- Concern about the extra time it would take to make physical activity recommendations

Figure 3-2. Barriers Practitioners Face in Recommending Physical Activity to Their Patients

Table 3-2. Oncology Nurse–Related Barriers and Strategies for Promoting Physical Activity

Barrier	Examples	Suggested Nursing Strategies
Personal beliefs and behaviors	Lack of importance placed on physical activity as compared to other healthcare interventions. Oncology nurses may therefore neglect to recommend physical activity to survivors. This is especially true when physical activity is not an important part of nurses' own lives. Oncologists also have been found to neglect recommending activity to survivors because of a lack of importance placed on this health parameter.	Maintain a positive attitude about physical activity. Participate in daily physical activity and create one's own activity program. The more positive a nurse is about physical activity and the more a nurse participates in physical activity, the more likely that nurse is to recommend activity to survivors. Encourage physician colleagues and oncology team members to serve as role models for physical activity.
	The belief that if survivors are not currently engaged in physical activity, then they are not interested in pursuing activity programs	Initiate the topic of physical activity during conversations with survivors and families. Have resources on physical activity available to survivors. Survivors are interested in learning about physical activity a good portion of the time.
Knowledge gap	Failure to make recommendations about physical activities due to lack of comfort, even when assessing for physical activities	Request or conduct organizational training programs on how to discuss physical activity with survivors and families.

(Continued on next page)

Table 3-2. Oncology Nurse–Related Barriers and Strategies for Promoting Physical Activity *(Continued)*

Barrier	Examples	Suggested Nursing Strategies
Knowledge gap *(cont.)*	Lack of comfort making physical activity recommendations due to a lack of knowledge related to evidence and best practices related to physical activity with cancer survivors; not understanding the effectiveness of physical activity on cancer survivors	Consult with physical therapy and occupational therapy to ensure safe activity programs for debilitated survivors or those with special considerations (see Chapters 12 and 13). Participate in evidence-based education activities that support physical activity in cancer survivors, such as journal clubs, continuing education from professional organizations, and self-learning through reputable online resources (e.g., Oncology Nursing Society, American College of Sports Medicine, National Comprehensive Cancer Network).
	Fear of harming survivors or of legal ramifications should injury occur during recommended physical activities	Maintain proficiency in physical activity and cancer survivorship. Create educational programs for oncology nurses and other professionals. Conduct education programs in collaboration with physical and occupational therapists, exercise physiologists, and rehabilitation specialists to ensure best practices and current evidence are met.
Lack of organizational support or structure	Lack of appropriate physical activity resources to use with survivors; existing resources are often not appropriately defined or specific enough and may not be readily available to staff members	Involve oncology nurses and oncology team members in developing evidence-based protocols and system processes to support physical activity recommendations and survivor adherence. Guidelines and resources should be developed based on current evidence and specific enough to support both survivors' and nurses' needs.
	Concerns about cost when approached about resources for survivors' physical activity suggestions and interventions	Create educational programs for oncology professionals that take costs and reimbursement into consideration. Measure cost savings through decreased use of oncology and healthcare services associated with physical activity.

(Continued on next page)

Table 3-2. Oncology Nurse–Related Barriers and Strategies for Promoting Physical Activity *(Continued)*

Barrier	Examples	Suggested Nursing Strategies
Lack of organizational support or structure *(cont.)*	Absence of protocols or daily systematic approach to recommending physical activity during patient and family encounters	Create protocols for referral to physical and occupational therapists, exercise physiologists, and exercise professionals.
Lack of time to address physical activity and exercise	Lack of time during survivor interactions and appointments for recommending physical activity	Incorporate assessment parameters related to physical activity during all survivor encounters.

Note. Based on information from Bakhshi et al., 2015; Haas, 2011; James-Martin et al., 2014; Karvinen et al., 2012; Keogh et al., 2014; Sander et al., 2012; Schmitz et al., 2010.

Application to Oncology Nursing Practice

1. Obtain a copy of the physical activity guidelines that are given to cancer survivors upon discharge from your cancer center. Compare this copy with the physical activities listed for cancer survivors receiving outpatient treatment. Note the similarities and differences.
2. Collaborate with physical and occupational therapists, as well as the oncology team, to create inpatient and outpatient guidelines for physical activities appropriate for cancer survivors. Search the literature and reputable websites to confirm your choices. Use your organization's policy and procedure process to put the guidelines into practice.
3. Join your oncology center's health and wellness committee. Work to develop simple physical activity programs for staff to follow.
4. Obtain a list of health clubs, walking trails, and other activity venues that cancer survivors can use.
5. Track your own physical activity using an electronic app or other tracking method (e.g., manual logging). Evaluate your activity choices and frequency.

Summary

Both barriers and opportunities exist for cancer survivors who want to become physically active. Oncology nurses, too, face similar barriers and opportunities in their personal and professional lives. Learning what motivates and encourages people to be active is an important part of oncology care. Cancer survivors desire information and support about physical activity, and oncology nurses can provide this support at every encounter. Organizations can incorporate physical activity questions into their patient assessments, provide safe areas for ambulation, and encourage interprofessional collaboration to create activity programs for staff and patients alike.

Case Study 1

S.M. is a 56-year-old patient at the infusion center following a colon resection. He is in his second month of active chemotherapy treatment. S.M. lives in a rural area and has not been educated on the benefits of physical activity nor how to be physically active. S.M. has a devoted wife who is often with him during his treatments. He also is close to his nurse, Jamie. Jamie and S.M. often talk about their love of walking outside. When talking with him and his wife, Jamie asks if they have been walking lately. His wife says she has been making him stay in bed all day and even brings him his meals because he is "just too sick to do anything else." S.M. complains of severe fatigue; he also says the chemotherapy makes him sick to his stomach, and he often doesn't feel like going outside.

Initial Exercise Prescription
- Begin with education about how physical activity can help with fatigue.
- Include S.M.'s wife in treatment and praise her for careful attention to S.M.'s needs; encourage them to walk together to the kitchen for meals.
- Address and bring to attention the physical activities S.M. performs, such as personal hygiene, and how to pace those activities throughout the day.
- On the next visit, follow up with S.M. and his wife to evaluate their physical activity program.

Case Study 2

S.W. has been an oncology nurse for two years and recently read an article on physical activity and its benefits to patients with cancer. She recognizes the need for increased interest by the staff in recommending physical activity to their patients. After a staff meeting, a group of interested unit staff volunteer to make a plan to increase the frequency of physical activity recommendations on their unit.

After talking with the staff, the group finds and addresses barriers as follows:
- Nursing staff is educated on the importance of physical activity for themselves and the availability of free classes at the hospital's employee gym.
- The original article S.W. had read is introduced to the staff, who read it and complete the post-test.
- The unit staff begins a physical activity club on the unit three days a week and a sneaker club for any patients who can ambulate.
- In this club, the patients experiencing symptoms such as fatigue and who meet criteria for the class meet for 30 minutes to learn from the nursing staff about the importance of physical activity and how it can benefit them. They then earn a sneaker sticker for every lap or short-term goal they achieve.
- The physical therapists are invited to demonstrate exercises, thus promoting interdepartmental collegiality.

References

Adams, A.K., Scott, J.R., Prince, R., & Williamson, A. (2014). Using community advisory boards to reduce environmental barriers to health in American Indian communities, Wisconsin, 2007–2012. *Preventing Chronic Disease, 11,* E160. Retrieved from http://www.cdc.gov/pcd/issues/2014/pdf/14_0014.pdf

Arroyave, W.D., Clipp, E.C., Miller, P.E., Jones, L.W., Ward, D.S., Bonner, M.J., ... Demark-Wahnefried, W. (2008). Childhood cancer survivors' perceived barriers to improving exercise and dietary behaviors. *Oncology Nursing Forum, 35,* 121–130. doi:10.1188/08.ONF.121-130

Bakhshi, S., Sun, F., Murrells, T., & While, A. (2015). Nurses' health behaviours and physical activity-related health-promotion practices. *British Journal of Community Nursing, 20,* 289–296. doi:10.12968/bjcn.2015.20.6.289

Bandura, A. (1997). Self-efficacy. *Harvard Mental Health Letter, 13*(9), 4–6.

Barber, F.D. (2013). Effects of social support on physical activity, self-efficacy, and quality of life in adult cancer survivors and their caregivers. *Oncology Nursing Forum, 40,* 481–489. doi:10.1188/13.ONF.481-489

Blaney, J.M., Lowe-Strong, A., Rankin-Watt, J., Campbell, A., & Gracey, J.H. (2013). Cancer survivors' exercise barriers, facilitators and preferences in the context of fatigue, quality of life and physical activity participation: A questionnaire–survey. *Psycho-Oncology, 22,* 186–194. doi:10.1002/pon.2072

Brant, J.M., & Wickham, R. (Eds.). (2013). *Statement on the scope and standards of oncology nursing practice: Generalist and advanced practice.* Pittsburgh, PA: Oncology Nursing Society.

Centers for Disease Control and Prevention. (2012). Trends in adults receiving a recommendation for exercise or other physical activity from a physician or other health professional. Retrieved from http://www.cdc.gov/nchs/data/databriefs/db86.htm

Fessele, K., Yendro, S., & Mallory, G. (2014). Setting the bar: Developing quality measures and education programs to define evidence-based, patient-centered, high-quality care. *Clinical Journal of Oncology Nursing, 18*(Suppl.), 7–11. doi:10.1188/14.CJON.S2.7-11

Forbes, C.C., Blanchard, C.M., Mummery, W.K., & Courneya, K.S. (2014). A comparison of physical activity correlates across breast, prostate, and colorectal cancer survivors in Nova Scotia, Canada. *Supportive Care in Cancer, 22,* 891–903. doi:10.1007/s00520-013-2045-7

Gho, S.A., Munro, B.J., Jones, S.C., & Steele, J.R. (2014). Exercise bra discomfort is associated with insufficient exercise levels among Australian women treated for breast cancer. *Supportive Care in Cancer, 22,* 721–729. doi:10.1007/s00520-013-2027-9

Haas, B.K. (2011). Fatigue, self-efficacy, physical activity, and quality of life in women with breast cancer. *Cancer Nursing, 34,* 322–334. doi:10.1097/NCC.0b013e3181f9a300

James-Martin, G., Koczwara, B., Smith, E.L., & Miller, M.D. (2014). Information needs of cancer patients and survivors regarding diet, exercise and weight management: A qualitative study. *European Journal of Cancer Care, 23,* 340–348. doi:10.1111/ecc.12159

Karvinen, K.H., McGourty, S., Parent, T., & Walker, P.R. (2012). Physical activity promotion among oncology nurses. *Cancer Nursing, 35,* E41–E48. doi:10.1097/NCC.0b013e31822d9081

Keogh, J.W., Patel, A., MacLeod, R.D., & Masters, J. (2014). Perceived barriers and facilitators to physical activity in men with prostate cancer: Possible influence of androgen deprivation therapy. *European Journal of Cancer Care, 23,* 263–273. doi:10.1111/ecc.12141

Olson, E.A., Mullen, S.P., Rogers, L.Q., Courneya, K.S., Verhulst, S., & McAuley, E. (2014). Meeting physical activity guidelines in rural breast cancer survivors. *American Journal of Health Behavior, 38,* 890–899. doi:10.5993/AJHB.38.6.11

Sander, A.P., Wilson, J., Izzo, N., Mountford, S.A., & Hayes, K.W. (2012). Factors that affect decisions about physical activity and exercise in survivors of breast cancer: A qualitative study. *Physical Therapy, 92,* 525–536. doi:10.2522/ptj.20110115

Schmitz, K.H., Courneya, K.S., Matthews, C., Demark-Wahnefried, W., Galvão, D., Pinto, B.M., ... Schwartz, A.L. (2010). American College of Sports Medicine roundtable on exercise guidelines for cancer survivors. *Medicine and Science in Sports and Exercise, 42*, 1409–1422. doi:10.1249/MSS.0b013e3181e0c112

Spector, D., Battaglini, C., & Groff, D. (2013). Perceived exercise barriers and facilitators among ethnically diverse breast cancer survivors. *Oncology Nursing Forum, 40*, 472–480. doi:10.1188/13.ONF.472-480

CHAPTER 4

FITT Principle for Physical Activity

Jeannette Q. Lee, PT, PhD

Introduction

Current evidence supports the importance of physical activity and exercise in cancer survivorship (Courneya & Friedenreich, 2001; Schmitz et al., 2010). Although exercise is a subset of physical activity, physical activity and exercise are different by definition (Durstine et al., 2009).

Physical activity is body movement that is produced by the contraction of skeletal muscles, resulting in significantly increased energy expenditure. Metabolic equivalent of tasks (METs) measure this energy expenditure. Table 4-1 lists the METs for various physical activities. Examples of physical activity include household physical activity (e.g., sweeping, scrubbing, vacuuming), workplace physical activity (e.g., lifting boxes, walking up and down stairs), and lifestyle physical activity (e.g., gardening).

Exercise, on the other hand, is a subset of physical activity that is planned, structured, and repetitive. Its purpose is to improve or maintain at least one aspect of physical fitness (e.g., muscular strength, muscular endurance, flexibility, cardiovascular endurance, body composition). Examples of exercise include walking on a treadmill or around the neighborhood for a set amount of time; swimming a set number of laps; practicing yoga, Pilates, or tai chi; and resistance training with elastic bands.

Researchers and fitness professionals use a specific framework for deciding the frequency, intensity, time, and type of physical activity and exercise. This is known as the FITT principle (or formula). This chapter will explore exercise as a

Table 4-1. Metabolic Equivalent of Tasks (METs) Associated With Selected Physical Activities

Category	Examples of Activities	METs
Household	Light	
	• Cleaning, sweeping	2.3
	• Washing dishes, clearing dishes from table	2.5
	Moderate	
	• Heavy or major cleaning (e.g., washing windows)	3.3
	• Kitchen activity, general (e.g., cooking, cleaning up)	3.5
	Vigorous	
	• Scrubbing floors, scrubbing bathroom	6.5
	• Carrying groceries upstairs	7.5
	• Moving boxes or furniture upstairs	9.0
Transportation	Light	
	• Riding in a car, bus, or train	1.3
	• Walking (1.7 mph) on level ground	2.3
	Moderate	
	• Walking (3 mph)	3.3
	• Bicycling (< 10 mph)	4.0
	Vigorous	
	• Climbing hills	6.3
	• Running (5 mph)	8.3
Occupation	Light	
	• Sitting tasks (e.g., writing, typing)	1.5
	• Cooking	2.5
	• Carpentry (general, light)	2.5
	Moderate	
	• Standing tasks (e.g., assembling, filing)	3.0
	• Electrical work (e.g., hooking up wires, splicing)	3.3
	• Farming (e.g., feeding animals, harvesting crops)	4.8
	Vigorous	
	• Shoveling, digging ditches	7.8
	• Using heavy power tools (e.g., jackhammers, drills)	8.0
Sports	Light	
	• Billiards	2.5
	• Playing catch (e.g., football, baseball)	2.5

(Continued on next page)

Table 4-1. Metabolic Equivalent of Tasks (METs) Associated With Selected Physical Activities *(Continued)*

Category	Examples of Activities	METs
Sports *(cont.)*	Moderate	
	• Bowling	3.8
	• Basketball (shooting hoops)	4.5
	• Golf (walking, pulling clubs)	5.3
	Vigorous	
	• Tennis	7.3
	• Basketball (game)	8.0
Recreation	Light	
	• Playing board games (sitting)	1.5
	• Playing musical instrument	2.0
	• Darts	2.5
	Moderate	
	• Fishing	3.5
	• Ballet or jazz dancing (class or rehearsal)	5.0
	• Hiking at a normal pace	5.3
	Vigorous	
	• Horseback riding (canter or gallop)	7.3
	• Rollerblading, in-line skating (9 mph)	7.5
	• General dancing (e.g., disco, folk, line dancing)	7.8
Exercise	Light	
	• Activity-promoting video games (e.g., Wii Fit™)	2.3
	• Balance, yoga, stretching	2.3
	• Walking (2.5 mph)	2.9
	Moderate	
	• Calisthenics	3.5
	• Stationary bicycle	4.8
	• Water aerobics, water exercise	5.3
	Vigorous	
	• Line dancing	7.8
	• Circuit training	8.0
	• Rowing, stationary	8.5

Note. Based on information from Ainsworth et al., 2011.

subcategory of physical activity and introduce the FITT principle to create and evaluate physical activity and exercise programs for cancer survivors. Oncology nurses can apply the FITT principle when recommending physical activity and exercise to their patients. This chapter's content is supported in the Oncology Nursing Society's *Statement on the Scope and Standards of Oncology Nursing Practice: Generalist and Advanced Practice* (Brant & Wickham, 2013) (see Figure 4-1) and the National Comprehensive Cancer Network® (NCCN®) guidelines (Ligibel & Denlinger, 2013; NCCN, 2015).

Standard I. Assessment
• Use appropriate evidence-based assessment techniques and instruments in collecting data, including valid and reliable instruments that assess the high-incidence problem areas (e.g., distress thermometer).

Standard II. Diagnosis
• Use evidence-based research to formulate the plan of care.

Standard III. Outcome Identification
• Ensure that expected outcomes are realistic in relation to the patient's present and potential capabilities.
• Design expected outcomes to maximize the patient's functional abilities.
• Assign a realistic time period for expected outcomes for achievement or reevaluation and be aware of the timing of side effects and normal physiologic events associated with cancer treatment and align expected outcomes accordingly.

Standard IV. Planning
• Incorporate appropriate preventive, therapeutic, rehabilitative, and palliative nursing actions into each phase of the plan of care along the cancer trajectory.
• Include individualized physical, psychological, and social interventions in the plan of care that are
  – Supported by current evidence-based research and practice
  – Designed to achieve the stated outcomes
  – Prioritized according to the patient's needs and preferences
  – Supportive of diversity awareness

Standard V. Implementation
• Use evidence-based research to guide implementation of interventions.

Standard VI. Evaluation
• Maintain a systematic and ongoing evaluation process.
• Collect evaluation data from all pertinent sources.
• Compare actual findings to expected findings.

Figure 4-1. Standards Applicable to Using the FITT Principle for Physical Activity and Exercise

---

Note. From *Statement on the Scope and Standards of Oncology Nursing Practice: Generalist and Advanced Practice,* by J.M. Brant and R. Wickham (Eds.), 2013, Pittsburgh, PA: Oncology Nursing Society. Copyright 2013 by Oncology Nursing Society. Adapted with permission.

Benefits of Physical Activity and Exercise in Cancer Survivors

Both physical activity and exercise are positively correlated to overall fitness and health-related quality of life (Bize, Johnson, & Plotnikoff, 2007; Caspersen, Powell, & Christenson, 1985). As discussed in Chapter 2, extensive research supports the benefits of physical activity in cancer survivors. Although cancer survivors may be encouraged to participate in physical activities and activities of daily living, exercise recommendations may not be provided. This could be because healthcare professionals, oncology nurses, and cancer survivors may mistakenly believe that exercise can be harmful during or after cancer treatment. Table 4-2 lists common myths and realities associated with exercise in cancer survivors.

Table 4-2. Myths and Realities of Exercise in Cancer Survivors

Myth	Reality
Exercising is too difficult for cancer survivors.	Exercise is important throughout cancer care. One or more of the exercise FITT principles may be modified (e.g., intensity) to assist with safe participation in exercise.
Exercise can cause injuries such as broken bones.	Physical activity, including weight-bearing activities such as walking, is important to promote bone tensile strength (see Chapter 12).
Side effects from treatment (e.g., dizziness) can cause falls.	Exercise and physical activity promote balance and coordination. Individuals can minimize falls by walking on flat surfaces, wearing supportive shoes, and carrying a cell phone or medical alert pendant; if an individual is at risk for falls, referrals for a balance program may be needed.
It is better to rest to conserve energy, especially if nauseated, fatigued, or in pain.	Immobility presents a formidable hazard, resulting in debilitation, falls, and injury. Individuals may benefit from small, frequent doses of physical activity when fatigued, nauseated, or in pain (see Chapter 8). • Stand up periodically and stretch. • Take deep breaths. • Sit and perform stretches. • Walk to the kitchen or bathroom. • Perform personal hygiene (e.g., wash face, brush teeth).
Lymphedema will worsen with exercise.	Physical activity and exercise can help alleviate lymphedema symptoms. Moreover, lymph flow has been shown to increase with exercise (see Chapter 12).
Exercise can only take place in the gym.	Individuals can get the benefits of exercise even at home. Walking is great exercise, and many household activities may help maintain overall fitness.

Physical activity and exercise provide many physical and emotional benefits for cancer survivors, such as the following (Bergenthal et al., 2014; Capozzi, Nishimura, McNeely, Lau, & Culos-Reed, 2015; Chan, McCarthy, Devenish, Sullivan, & Chan, 2015; Meneses-Echávez, González-Jiménez, & Ramírez-Vélez, 2015; Mishra, Scherer, Snyder, Geigle, & Gotay, 2014, 2015):

- Improved aerobic fitness
- Improved flexibility and range of motion
- Improved circulation
- Improved muscle strength
- Reduced fatigue
- Maintenance of bone density
- Weight management
- Improved self-esteem
- Reduced feelings of anxiety or depression
- Increased relaxation
- Transitioning focus from being ill to getting better

During the medical management of cancer, exercise can improve tolerance to cancer treatment, mediate side effects, and improve sleep. Following treatment, exercise can improve mobility, strength, and endurance.

For individuals who are very active in sports or who exercise daily, physical activity alone may not provide any additional health benefits. For many people, a combination of physical activity and exercise seems to be the easiest to maintain over time. During periods of fatigue, exercise may become less intense and frequent, and physical activities may become more frequent. It is important for cancer survivors to find activities that they enjoy and do them regularly.

Principles of Exercise Training

Understanding exercise training principles helps oncology nurses educate cancer survivors on the expected outcomes of regular physical activity and exercise. These principles also help oncology nurses modify physical activity and exercise programs when survivors experience improvement in their physical fitness and are ready to change their program (Winters-Stone, Neill, & Campbell, 2014).

The FITT Principle

The accepted method for organizing and planning physical activity and exercise is with the FITT principle: frequency, intensity, time, and type (see Table 4-3). Each component of the FITT principle can be adjusted to be easier or more challenging, depending on an individual's fitness level, time availability, and fitness goals. Ideally, cancer survivors should be physically active every day; exercise may or may not be a part of that daily physical activity.

Table 4-3. FITT Principle

FITT Principle	Description	Measurement
Frequency	How often one exercises	Number of days per week
Intensity	How hard one exercises	The intensity of exercise can be measured by various relative intensity or absolute intensity methods. *Relative intensity* is the level of effort required by an individual to perform an activity. *Absolute intensity* is the amount of energy that an individual's body uses per minute of activity. **Talk test**—Individual tries to carry on a conversation or sing while exercising. • Low intensity: Individual is able to sing while exercising. • Moderate intensity: Individual is challenged but can carry on a conversation and is not out of breath. • High intensity: Individual is unable to carry on a conversation or is out of breath. The intensity may be too high and should be lowered. **Target heart rate**—Heart rate is measured in beats per minute. Heart rate can be measured in several ways: • Use the Karvonen formula to calculate target heart rate by calculating the individual's age and resting heart rate (see Chapters 6 and 7). • Wear a heart rate monitor that displays heart rate while exercising. • Palpate the radial or carotid artery for 10 seconds and multiply that number by 6 to calculate beats/minute. When exercising, individuals should periodically check their heart rate to see if it is in their target zone. If their heart rate is too low or too high, then the intensity of the exercise can be modified. • Moderate intensity: Individual's heart rate is approximately 50%–70% of maximum heart rate (MHR). • Vigorous intensity: Individual's heart rate is approximately 70%–85% of MHR. **Rating of perceived exertion (RPE)**—RPE is a self-rating of effort or strain during exercise. The original version of the scale runs from 6–20, where 6 indicates no exertion and 20 represents maximum exertion.

(Continued on next page)

Table 4-3. FITT Principle *(Continued)*

FITT Principle	Description	Measurement
Intensity *(cont.)*		Another version of the scale runs from 0–10, where 0 indicates "no effort at all" and 10 indicates "very, very hard." Using the RPE scale method would be appropriate for individuals whose medication may affect their heart rate and how it responds to exercise. To view these scales, visit www.heartonline .org.au/media/DRL/Rating_of_perceived_exertion_-_Borg_scale.pdf.
Time	How long one exercises	Minutes of exercise
Type	What kind of exercise	Cardiovascular/aerobic Strength/resistance Flexibility

FITT—frequency, intensity, time, type

Note. Based on information from Centers for Disease Control and Prevention, 2015a, 2015b.

A well-balanced exercise program (see Figure 4-2) also incorporates relaxation and rest, which help to decrease the negative effects of chronic stress on the mind and body. During rest, energy continues to be expended but at a very low rate.

In regard to activity, cancer survivors should do the following (De Backer, Schep, Backx, Vreugdenhil, & Kuipers, 2009; NCCN, 2015; Schmitz et al., 2010):

- Be as active as possible (as health conditions allow).
- Avoid inactivity.
- Modify exercises (i.e., decrease exercise intensity) if they have known bone metastasis, and avoid activities linked to fracture risks (e.g., contact sports, climbing).
- Have increased supervision or complete exercise testing when beginning an exercise program if known cardiac conditions exist (Schmitz et al., 2010; U.S. Department of Health and Human Services [DHHS], 2008).

Exercise Guidelines for Cancer Survivors

Exercise guidelines are determined based on the type of exercise: cardiovascular/aerobic, strength/resistance, or flexibility. The exercise guidelines discussed in this chapter are based on the 2010 American College of Sports Medicine

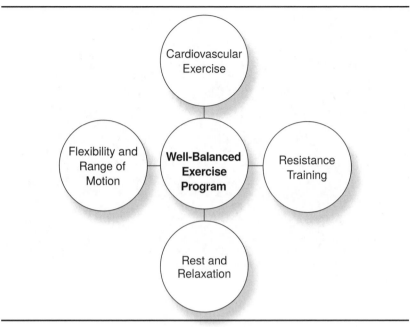

Figure 4-2. Components of a Well-Balanced Exercise Program

(ACSM) roundtable on exercise guidelines for cancer survivors and DHHS's *Physical Activity Guidelines Advisory Committee Report*.

Cardiovascular Exercise

Cardiovascular exercise tends to focus on larger muscle groups. A wide range of exercise protocols and regimens for survivors of many cancer types have been reported in the literature (Bergenthal et al., 2014; Fong et al., 2012; McNeely et al., 2006; Speck, Courneya, Mâsse, Duval, & Schmitz, 2010; Thorsen, Courneya, Stevinson, & Fosså, 2008). A one-size-fits-all program for cancer survivors is difficult to recommend because of the wide variety of cancer types and treatments.

Using the FITT principle, general guidelines for cardiovascular exercise are as follows (Schmitz et al., 2010; U.S. DHHS, 2008).

- Frequency: Three to five days per week is ideal. Individuals should not take two days off in a row.
- Intensity: Moderate or vigorous intensity (or a combination) is encouraged; intensity level can be assessed through the talk test, target heart rate, or Borg rating of perceived exertion (RPE) (see Table 4-3). Using the RPE scale method (Borg, 1982) would be appropriate for individuals whose medications may affect their heart rate and how it responds to exercise.

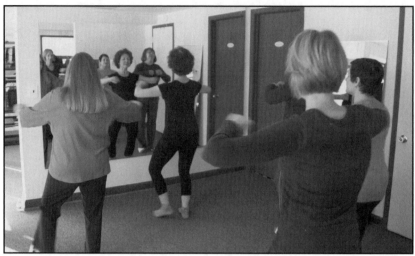

Dancing is an example of a moderate- to vigorous-intensity cardiovascular exercise that can be performed in a group setting.

- Time: A total of 150 minutes of moderate-intensity exercise or 75 minutes of vigorous-intensity exercise (or a combination) per week is recommended. Individuals should exercise for at least 20–30 continuous minutes per day but may start with multiple short bouts (e.g., 5–10 minutes) with rest intervals.
- Type: Walking and cycling (stationary or leisure) are excellent activities to start. Other examples of cardiovascular exercise are dancing, jogging, and swimming.

Strength/Resistance Exercise

Resistance training for cancer survivors can improve both muscular endurance and strength (Cheema, Gaul, Lane, & Singh, 2008; De Backer et al., 2009; Fong et al., 2012; Strasser, Steindorf, Wiskemann, & Ulrich, 2013). Resistance training also is important for strong bones and performance of daily activities.

Muscular strength can be measured by *one-repetition maximum* (1RM), defined as the maximum weight a person can lift only once in complete range of motion (Abernethy, Wilson, & Logan, 1995). Muscular strength also can be measured by 6RM or 7RM to estimate 1RM. Muscular endurance can be measured by the number of repetitions a person can lift of a certain weight in a given time.

Resistance training should start with a supervised program (for proper form) and at a low resistance, progressing in small increments, particularly if the individual is new to resistance training (Schmitz et al., 2010; U.S. DHHS, 2008).

Using the FITT principle, general guidelines for resistance exercise are as follows (Schmitz et al., 2010; U.S. DHHS, 2008):

- Frequency: Two to three times per week is ideal. Muscles need about 24–48 hours to recover between exercise sessions.
- Intensity: 25%–85% of 1RM, or 8–12 repetitions (or lower to start), is encouraged. Individuals should perform 1–2 sets for large muscle groups of the body, including both upper and lower extremities and trunk and back muscles.
- Time: Length of time varies depending on the number of reps and sets, but primarily five to nine large muscle group exercises can be completed in 10-minute increments.
- Type: Hand weights, elastic bands, gym equipment, and body weight are excellent resources for resistance training.

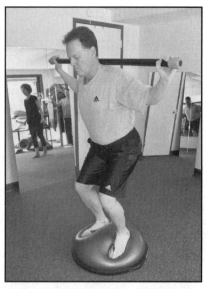

Resistance training can be combined with balance training for cancer survivors who are ready for more advanced activities.

Flexibility Exercise

Flexibility exercises stretch major muscle groups and tendons and are important for full range of motion and make it easier to perform activities of daily living. Range of motion may be especially problematic after surgery or radiation therapy. Although the breadth of flexibility exercises for cancer survivors reported in the literature is less than that of cardiovascular or resistance exercises, many benefits exist for individuals who perform flexibility exercises following cancer treatment (Schmitz et al., 2010; Speck et al., 2010).

Using the FITT principle, general guidelines for flexibility exercise are as follows (Schmitz et al., 2010; U.S. DHHS, 2008):

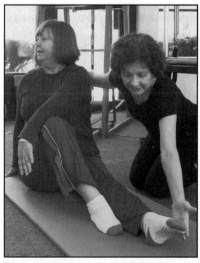

To ensure proper technique, flexibility training with guidance from an instructor can be helpful for cancer survivors just getting started.

- Frequency: At least two times per week is encouraged (after warm-up or cooldown); daily would be optimal.
- Intensity: Flexibility exercises should be low intensity, gentle, and in the pain-free range of motion.
- Time: Each stretch should be held 20–30 seconds to the point of tightness or slight discomfort only. Repeat each stretch two to four times.
- Type: Flexibility exercises can consist of gently stretching large muscle groups and tendons; stretches can be done while standing or seated against a wall.

Oncology Nursing Recommendations for Beginning an Exercise Program

Cancer survivors may need help from their oncology nurse on how to get started with a physical activity or exercise program. Oncology nurses can help cancer survivors prepare for physical activity and exercise programs. The steps that survivors should take before, during, and after being physically active or exercising are outlined in the next few sections. Writing down these steps can help cancer survivors be safe and effective when exercising. Evidence-based guidelines for cancer-specific and side effect–specific physical activities and exercises are presented in Chapters 8–13.

Before the Exercise Program

- Consult with your oncology team to determine the frequency, intensity, type, and time of exercise appropriate for the cancer survivor. There may be restrictions (e.g., not lifting more than five pounds, being mindful of balance issues) that individuals need to follow.
- Tailor physical activity/exercise sessions based on chemotherapy treatment schedules. Decrease the intensity of exercise during chemotherapy treatment if needed and advise survivors to perform physical activities only. For low-intensity activities, offer restorative/resting yoga, stretching, or meditation. Survivors should avoid swimming pools during radiation treatments and wear a mask when exercising in a group if blood counts are low.
- Choose physical activities and exercises that fit with the survivor's current lifestyle, routine, and personal preferences.
  - Would the individual prefer to exercise alone, or would being in a group help motivate him or her?
  - Is it easier for the cancer survivor to exercise in the morning or later in the afternoon?
  - Does the survivor prefer DVDs or video streaming of physical activity and exercises or "live" exercise sessions?

During the Exercise Program

- "Start low; progress slow." This adage is especially applicable if the cancer survivor was previously sedentary or is new to participation in regular physical activity or exercise. Even people who were very active prior to their cancer diagnosis might experience reductions in physical fitness because of cancer treatment, so starting slow and then building up to more exercises or newer activities is important to prevent injuries and build tolerance. Exercise tolerance may vary from session to session, particularly after an operation or during treatment.
- Warm up before exercising. Warming up the large muscle groups may help to reduce risk of injury (Fradkin, Gabbe, & Cameron, 2006). Warm-up exercises include walking slowly in place or on a treadmill, pedaling slowly on an exercise bicycle, and moving arms and legs in a rhythmic motion. Warm-up exercises require about 5–10 minutes (for a 60-minute exercise session) to gradually increase the heart rate and warm up the muscles. A rule of thumb is the warm-up and cooldown should each be about 15% of the time of the entire exercise session. The pace can be increased until the person feels warm.
- Stop immediately if adverse events are experienced, such as shortness of breath, chest pain, dizziness, irregular heartbeat, or any increased joint or limb pain. If these symptoms persist, a consultation with the oncology team is warranted.
- Wear comfortable clothes and proper footwear during exercise. Proper footwear is important, especially if the cancer survivor has peripheral neuropathy or decreased sensation in the feet from cancer treatments. When exercising in a

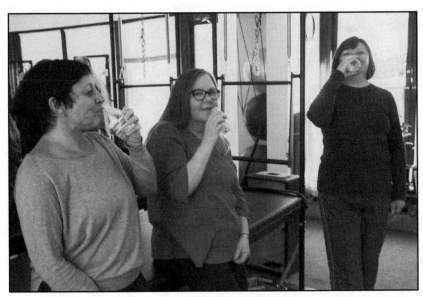

Maintain hydration by drinking water before, during, and after physical activity and exercise.

group setting, individuals should bring their own mat, towel, and water bottle to promote personal hygiene.

- Stay hydrated throughout the exercise session, taking time every few minutes for a sip of water. Hydration is important during chemotherapy and radiation therapy. Additional fluids may be required based on humidity levels and exercise intensity.
- Measure heart rate and intensity during the exercise session. Teach the cancer survivor how to measure heart rate and RPE or use the talk test (see Table 4-3); calculate their target heart rate and target heart rate zone (see Chapters 6 and 7).
- Teach cancer survivors about the effects their medications and treatments may have on muscle fatigue, cramping, or discomfort while exercising. Teach survivors how to recognize these feelings and how to prevent or treat them. To prevent muscle distress, encourage the person to remember which exercises or activities cause distress and to avoid them. To treat these effects, survivors should stop the exercise or activity gradually and stretch, hydrate, and resume when feeling better.

After the Exercise Program

- Cool down after exercise. Cooling down the large muscle groups reduces stress on the heart and muscles. In contrast to the warm-up, the cooldown gradually decreases the heart rate and relaxes the muscles. Cooldown exercises require about 5–10 minutes (for a 60-minute exercise session). Activities for warming up also may be used for cooling down. A rule of thumb is the warm-up and cooldown should be about 30% of the time of the entire exercise session.

Application to Oncology Nursing Practice

1. Obtain a copy of your oncology center's list of physical activities and exercises for cancer survivors. If one is not available, use this guidebook to begin creating a useful list. Evaluate your center's program against the components in Figure 4-2. Determine the strengths and weaknesses of your center's program. Collaborate with the oncology team to strengthen and balance your physical activity and exercise programs for cancer survivors.
2. Review the guidelines for cardiovascular exercise, strength/resistance exercise, and flexibility exercise. Talk with the cancer survivor; create an exercise program using the guidelines and activities from Table 4-1.
3. Create an exercise program for yourself using the guidelines for cardiovascular exercise, strength/resistance exercise, and flexibility exercise. Incorporate activities from Table 4-1.

4. Compare and contrast the recommendations in the literature for patients beginning an exercise program with the recommendations put forth by your oncology center.

5. Refer to Table 4-3. Teach survivors how to measure their heart rate or use the talk test. Create take-home instructions for cancer survivors on how to calculate their target heart rate and target heart rate zones. Create an RPE form for survivors to use. Alternatively, use the charts for target heart rates in Table 4-4.

Table 4-4. Target Heart Rate Maximum Target Training Zones

Age	Approximate Maximum Heart Rate[a]	Maximum Target Training Zones[b] (beats per minute)					
	Heart Rate	60%	65%	70%	75%	80%	85%
20	200	120	130	140	150	160	170
25	195	117	127	137	146	156	166
30	190	114	124	133	143	152	166
35	185	111	120	130	139	148	157
40	180	108	117	126	135	144	153
45	175	105	114	123	131	140	149
50	170	102	111	119	128	136	145
55	165	99	107	116	124	132	140
60	160	96	104	112	120	128	136
65	155	93	101	109	116	124	132
70	150	90	98	105	113	120	128
75	145	87	94	102	109	116	123
80	140	84	91	98	105	112	119

[a] Approximate maximum heart rate is calculated by subtracting the patient's age from 220.

[b] Maximum target training zones are calculated by multiplying the maximum heart rate by a percentage.

Note. Based on information from American Heart Association, 2015.

Summary

Cancer survivors will ask their oncology nurse about getting started with exercise. The FITT principle helps individuals and nurses derive an exercise plan that is achievable, based on the individual's activity preferences.

Case Study 1

A.D. is a 65-year-old woman who has recently completed six courses of chemotherapy secondary to acute myeloid leukemia. She is a retired seamstress who lives in a split-level home with her husband and 11-year-old granddaughter. Prior to diagnosis, A.D. lived a relatively sedentary lifestyle; she prefers instead to stay at home and watch television. A.D. currently reports being easily fatigued. She is willing to increase her activity level but expresses some anxiety about engaging in physical activity and exercise. She does not enjoy exercising but would really like to feel "more energetic and less tired" (see Figure 4-3).

Relevant Laboratory Values
- Hematocrit: 33%
- Hemoglobin: 10 g/dl

Medical History
- Relatively unremarkable
- No significant risks for cardiovascular disease

Special Considerations
- A.D. was previously sedentary and reports that she does not enjoy exercising. Start out with activities that are relatively easy to incorporate into her lifestyle to encourage engagement and adherence.

Height/weight	• Height: 5'7" • Weight: 169 lbs • BMI: 26.5 • Overweight
Vitals	• Blood pressure: 123/82 mm Hg • Resting heart rate: 79 bpm • Respiratory rate: 18 breaths per minute • Temperature: 98.78°F (37.1°C)
Cardiopulmonary	• Cardiopulmonary screen within normal limits

Figure 4-3. Additional Patient Information

BMI—body mass index; bpm—beats per minute

- A.D. may be feeling fatigued after chemotherapy. Increasing physical activity is an effective strategy to alleviate cancer-related fatigue. Start with significantly shorter bouts of activity at a lower intensity and work toward a goal of 20–30 minutes of continuous activity at a moderate intensity. Find a sufficient challenge point for activity; for example, A.D. should be able to sing while performing activity.
- Consider A.D.'s lower-than-normal hematocrit and hemoglobin values. Care must be taken to incorporate rest intervals regularly and to monitor A.D.'s response to exercise, as the low hematocrit and hemoglobin levels may make A.D. more prone to shortness of breath or dizziness.

Sample Initial Exercise Prescription				
Exercise Type	Frequency	Intensity	Time	Type
Strength	1–3 times per week on alternating days	One set, 8–10 reps to start, with light weights	8–10 exercises addressing major muscle groups	Begin with body weight exercises and progress to free weights or machine weights as tolerance improves.
Cardiovascular	Start with 3 days per week and progress to 5 or more days per week.	Light to start (up to 50% maximum heart rate or Borg rating of perceived exertion [RPE] of 2–3/10) Individual should be able to talk during exercise without feeling out of breath. Progress to moderate physical exertion or 50%–70% maximum heart rate or RPE of 4/10.	Total of 150 minutes per week. Start with 5–10-minute bouts. Progress to 20–30 minutes of continued activity per day.	Begin with walking around the house and progress to stairs and hills as activity tolerance allows.
Flexibility	Start with 3 days per week and progress to 5 or more days per week.	To the point of resistance	5–10 minutes of stretching warm-up and cooldown with endurance activity Hold each stretch for 20–30 seconds.	Low-load prolonged positional or active stretching

Case Study 2

C.B. is a 44-year-old woman who is being treated with chemotherapy for breast cancer. She reports that she also will be receiving radiation therapy after the chemotherapy regimen has been completed. C.B. owns a local café and lives with her husband and 14-year-old son. She is a health-conscious woman and enjoys spending time gardening and working in her greenhouse. She was previously an avid mountain biker and would like to return to that activity.

C.B. has started noticing that she feels much weaker than before and feels stiffer as she goes about her day. Treatment with chemotherapy has resulted in persistent neuropathy, and the surgery on her right side has resulted in her right arm having slightly less range of motion than her left arm (see Figure 4-4).

Relevant Laboratory Values
- Hemoglobin: 13.2 g/dl
- White blood cell count: 2,600/mm³

Medical History
- Right breast lumpectomy
- Four lymph nodes removed

Special Considerations
- New treatment-related exercise concerns have presented for a formerly active patient. Mountain biking is an activity that requires stamina (cardiorespiratory fitness), muscular strength, flexibility, and balance. Refer to a physical therapist for evaluation.
- Because of neuropathy from chemotherapy, her ability to hold weights (if hands are affected) or alter her balance (if feet are affected) may be limited.
- The decreased range of motion of her shoulder may also prevent her from completing some exercises. Check for any signs and symptoms of lymphedema in her right arm.
- Because of these aforementioned issues, it would be best that the first several weeks of C.B.'s exercise regimen be supervised in order to monitor her response to exercise.

Height/weight	• Height: 5'8" • Weight: 149 lbs • BMI: 22.7 • Healthy weight
Vitals	• Blood pressure: 126/76 mm Hg • Resting heart rate: 74 bpm • Respiratory rate: 17 breaths per minute • Temperature: 98.6°F (37°C)
Cardiopulmonary	• Cardiovascular examination normal • Breath sounds normal bilaterally

Figure 4-4. Additional Patient Information

BMI—body mass index; bpm—beats per minute

Sample Initial Exercise Prescription				
Exercise Type	Frequency	Intensity	Time	Type
Strength	Twice weekly, with 1–2 days of rest between sessions	One set, 8–10 reps to start, with the lightest weights For upper extremity exercises, the individual would progress by the smallest increments after completing 2–3 sessions with the same weights and sets.	8–10 exercises addressing major muscle groups	Light weights with dumbbells or weight machine or low-resistance exercise bands Use of variable-resistance machines may be warranted if neuropathy is present on the hands, preventing individual from holding dumbbells or resistance bands.
Flexibility	At the end of each exercise session	Done gently, in the pain-free range of motion	Hold each stretch for 20–30 seconds to the point of tightness, repeating each stretch 2–4 times. Extra focus should be on gradually increasing range of motion on the right arm and shoulder.	Large muscle groups (e.g., shoulder, arm, chest, hamstrings, calf) in seated or standing position

Case Study 3

H.G. is a 63-year-old man with stage II prostate cancer. He will be finishing his radiation treatment within the next week and has expressed interest in becoming more physically active. H.G. works as an office manager and has been able to work part time during treatment. He plans on returning to work three days per week for the next few months to make time for doctors' appointments. H.G. is married and has two grown children and five grandchildren. He has reported fatigue and that it is harder for him to complete work-related tasks without tiring. He is not physically active but would like to be able to join his wife and grandchildren for bike rides and walks on local bike paths. H.G. reports that he is nervous because it has been so long since he has been active.

Relevant Laboratory Values
- Hemoglobin: 12 g/dl
- White blood cell count: 7,000/mm^3

Medical History
- Overweight
- Type II diabetes

Special Considerations
- Because H.G. is very deconditioned and unsure of himself, it is important to start with exercises and parameters in which he will be successful and build his confidence while beginning to build a foundation for more rigorous activity.
- As H.G. continues to progress, his exercise prescription may be increased to a vigorous intensity. However, he will achieve the recommended level of activity for his age with a moderate exercise program.
- Monitor H.G.'s diabetes and ensure blood sugar regulation.

Sample Initial Exercise Prescription				
Exercise Type	Frequency	Intensity	Time	Type
Strength and balance	Once per week	Body weight	20 minutes	Tai chi DVD for 20 minutes at home once a week
Cardio-vascular	3 times per week	Light to start (up to 50% maximum heart rate or RPE of 2–3/10) Individual should be able to easily talk during exercise without feeling out of breath.	15–20 minutes	Recumbent cycling or walking

(Continued on next page)

Sample Initial Exercise Prescription *(Continued)*				
Exercise Type	**Frequency**	**Intensity**	**Time**	**Type**
Flexibility	2–3 times per week	Low load to the point of resistance. Each stretch should be held for 20–30 seconds.	5–10 minutes of stretching warm-up and cooldown with aerobic exercise	Prolonged positional or active stretching
Sample Moderate Exercise Progression				
Strength	1–2 times per week	60%–70% of one repetition maximum (1RM), 8–12 reps, 1–2 sets	8–10 exercises addressing major muscle groups	Free weights, machines, resistance bands, or body weight
Cardio-vascular	3–5 times per week	Moderate physical exertion or 50%–70% maximum heart rate or RPE of 4/10	20–45 minutes	Recumbent cycling or walking
Flexibility	3–5 times per week	Low load to the point of resistance	5–10 minutes of stretching warm-up and cooldown with aerobic exercise	Prolonged positional or active stretching
Balance	Once per week	Progress to decreased base of support/need for external support from initial prescription.	20 minutes	Tai chi DVD for 20 minutes at home once a week
Sample Vigorous Exercise Progression				
Exercise Type	**Frequency**	**Intensity**	**Time**	**Type**
Strength	2–3 times per week	70%–80% of 1RM, 8–12 reps, 2–3 sets	8–10 exercises addressing major muscle groups	Free weights, machines, resistance bands, or body weight

(Continued on next page)

Sample Vigorous Exercise Progression *(Continued)*				
Exercise Type	Frequency	Intensity	Time	Type
Cardio-vascular	3–7 times per week	Somewhat hard to hard (50%–70% maximum heart rate or RPE of 4/10)	45–60 min-utes	Cycling or walking
Flexibility	Before and after exer-cise ses-sion (warm-up and cooldown)	Low load to point of resistance	5–10 minutes of stretching warm-up and cooldown with aerobic exercise	Prolonged positional or active stretching
Balance	1–2 times per week	Progress to decreased base of support/need for external sup-port from initial prescription	20 minutes	Tai chi DVD at home

The author would like to acknowledge Kara Tischer, PT, DPT, Kelly McCor-mick, PT, DPT, Betsy J. Becker, PT, DPT, CLT-LANA, and Lisa M. Bernardo, PhD, MPH, RN, CEP, CCET, for their contributions to the case studies.

References

Abernethy, P., Wilson, G., & Logan, P. (1995). Strength and power assessment. Issues, controver-sies, and challenges. *Sports Medicine, 19*, 401–417. doi:10.2165/00007256-199519060-00004

Ainsworth, B.E., Haskell, W.L., Herrmann, S.D., Meckes, N., Bassett, D.R., Jr., Tudor-Locke, C., ... Leon, A.S. (2011). 2011 compendium of physical activities: A second update of codes and MET values. *Medicine and Science in Sports and Exercise, 43*, 1575–1581. doi:10.1249/MSS.0b013e31821ece12

American Heart Association. (2015). Target heart rates. Retrieved from http://www.heart.org/HEARTORG/HealthyLiving/PhysicalActivity/FitnessBasics/Target-Heart-Rates_UCM_434341_Article.jsp#.V1g9QNIrKUk

Bergenthal, N., Will, A., Streckmann, F., Wolkewitz, K.D., Monsef, I., Engert, A., ... Skoetz, N. (2014). Aerobic physical exercise for adult patients with haematological malignancies. *Cochrane Database of Systematic Reviews, 2014*(11). doi:10.1002/14651858.cd009075.pub2

Bize, R., Johnson, J.A., & Plotnikoff, R.C. (2007). Physical activity level and health-related quality of life in the general adult population: A systematic review. *Preventive Medicine, 45*, 401–415. doi:10.1016/j.ypmed.2007.07.017

Borg, G.A.V. (1982). Psychophysical bases of perceived exertion. *Medicine and Science in Sports and Exercise, 14,* 377–381.

Brant, J.M., & Wickham, R. (Eds.). (2013). *Statement on the scope and standards of oncology nursing practice: Generalist and advanced practice.* Pittsburgh, PA: Oncology Nursing Society.

Capozzi, L.C., Nishimura, K.C., McNeely, M.L., Lau, H., & Culos-Reed, S.N. (2016). The impact of physical activity on health-related fitness and quality of life for patients with head and neck cancer: A systematic review. *British Journal of Sports Medicine, 50,* 325–338. doi:10.1136/bjsports-2015-094684

Caspersen, C.J., Powell, K.E., & Christenson, G.M. (1985). Physical activity, exercise, and physical fitness: Definitions and distinctions for health-related research. *Public Health Reports, 100,* 126–131.

Centers for Disease Control and Prevention. (2015a). Glossary of terms. Retrieved from http://www.cdc.gov/physicalactivity/basics/glossary

Centers for Disease Control and Prevention. (2015b). Target heart rate and estimated maximum heart rate. Retrieved from http://www.cdc.gov/physicalactivity/everyone/measuring/heartrate.html

Chan, R.J., McCarthy, A.L., Devenish, J., Sullivan, K.A., & Chan, A. (2015). Systematic review of pharmacologic and non-pharmacologic interventions to manage cognitive alterations after chemotherapy for breast cancer. *European Journal of Cancer, 51,* 437–450. doi:10.1016/j.ejca.2014.12.017

Cheema, B., Gaul, C.A., Lane, K., & Singh, M.A.F. (2008). Progressive resistance training in breast cancer: A systematic review of clinical trials. *Breast Cancer Research and Treatment, 109,* 9–26. doi:10.1007/s10549-007-9638-0

Courneya, K.S., & Friedenreich, C.M. (2001). Framework PEACE: An organizational model for examining physical exercise across the cancer experience. *Annals of Behavioral Medicine, 23,* 263–272. doi:10.1207/S15324796ABM2304_5

De Backer, I.C., Schep, G., Backx, F.J., Vreugdenhil, G., & Kuipers, H. (2009). Resistance training in cancer survivors: A systematic review. *International Journal of Sports Medicine, 30,* 703–712. doi:10.1055/s-0029-1225330

Durstine, J.L., Peel, J.B., LaMonte, M.J., Keteyian, S.J., Fletcher, E., & Moore, G.E. (2009). Exercise is medicine. In J.L. Durstine, G. Moore, P. Painter, & S.O. Roberts (Eds.), *ACSM's exercise management for persons with chronic diseases and disabilities* (3rd ed., pp. 21–30). Champaign, IL: Human Kinetics.

Fong, D.Y., Ho, J.W., Hui, B.P., Lee, A.M., Macfarlane, D.J., Leung, S.S., ... Cheng, K.K. (2012). Physical activity for cancer survivors: Meta-analysis of randomised controlled trials. *BMJ, 344,* E70. doi:10.1136/bmj.e70

Fradkin, A.J., Gabbe, B.J., & Cameron, P.A. (2006). Does warming up prevent injury in sport? *Journal of Science and Medicine in Sport, 9,* 214–220. doi:10.1016/j.jsams.2006.03.026

Ligibel, J.A., & Denlinger, C.S. (2013). New NCCN guidelines for survivorship care. *Journal of the National Comprehensive Cancer Network, 11*(Suppl. 5), 640–644.

McNeely, M.L., Campbell, K.L., Rowe, B.H., Klassen, T.P., Mackey, J.R., & Courneya, K.S. (2006). Effects of exercise on breast cancer patients and survivors: A systematic review and meta-analysis. *Canadian Medical Association Journal, 175,* 34–41. doi:10.1503/cmaj.051073

Meneses-Echávez, J.F., González-Jiménez, E., & Ramírez-Vélez, R. (2015). Supervised exercise reduces cancer-related fatigue: A systematic review. *Journal of Physiotherapy, 61,* 3–9. doi:10.1016/j.jphys.2014.08.019

Mishra, S.I., Scherer, R.W., Snyder, C., Geigle, P., & Gotay, C. (2014). Are exercise programs effective for improving health-related quality of life among cancer survivors? A systematic review and meta-analysis [Online exclusive]. *Oncology Nursing Forum, 41,* E326–E342. doi:10.1188/14.ONF.E326-E342

Mishra, S.I., Scherer, R.W., Snyder, C., Geigle, P., & Gotay, C. (2015). The effectiveness of exercise interventions for improving health-related quality of life from diagnosis through active cancer treatment [Online exclusive]. *Oncology Nursing Forum, 42,* E33–E53. doi:10.1188/15.ONF.E33-E53

National Comprehensive Cancer Network. (2015). *NCCN Clinical Practice Guidelines in Oncology (NCCN Guidelines®): Cancer survivorship* [v.2.2015]. Retrieved from https://www.nccn.org/professionals/physician_gls/f_guidelines.asp#supportive

Schmitz, K.H., Courneya, K.S., Matthews, C., Demark-Wahnefried, W., Galvão, D.A., Pinto, B.M., ... Schwartz, A.L. (2010). American College of Sports Medicine roundtable on exercise guidelines for cancer survivors. *Medicine and Science in Sports and Exercise, 42,* 1409–1426. doi:10.1249/MSS.0b013e3181e0c112

Speck, R.M., Courneya, K.S., Mâsse, L.C., Duval, S., & Schmitz, K.H. (2010). An update of controlled physical activity trials in cancer survivors: A systematic review and meta-analysis. *Journal of Cancer Survivorship Research, 4,* 87–100. doi:10.1007/s11764-009-0110-5

Strasser, B., Steindorf, K., Wiskemann, J., & Ulrich, C. (2013). Impact of resistance training in cancer survivors: A meta-analysis. *Medicine and Science in Sports and Exercise, 45,* 2080–2090. doi:10.1249/MSS.0b013e31829a3b63

Thorsen, L., Courneya, K.S., Stevinson, C., & Fosså, S.D. (2008). A systematic review of physical activity in prostate cancer survivors: Outcomes, prevalence, and determinants. *Supportive Care in Cancer, 16,* 987–997. doi:10.1007/s00520-008-0411-7

U.S. Department of Health and Human Services. (2008). *Physical activity guidelines advisory committee report, 2008.* Washington, DC: Author.

Winters-Stone, K.M., Neill, S.E., & Campbell, K.L. (2014). Attention to principles of exercise training: A review of exercise studies for survivors of cancers other than breast. *British Journal of Sports Medicine, 48,* 987–995. doi:10.1136/bjsports-2012-091732

CHAPTER 5

Assessing Readiness for Physical Activity

Frances Westlake, PT, DPT, NCS, Alaina Newell, PT, DPT, WCS, CLT-LANA, and Betsy J. Becker, PT, DPT, CLT-LANA

Introduction

Engaging in physical activity and exercise is a behavior that is based on desire and motivation. Changing one's behavior to participate in physical activity and exercise and make it a habit is no small task. This chapter focuses on motivation and readiness for behavior change with evidence from a range of frameworks. Methods to measure the stages of readiness for behavior change and strategies to promote change based on the stage of readiness are addressed. This chapter's content is supported in the Oncology Nursing Society's *Statement on the Scope and Standards of Oncology Nursing Practice: Generalist and Advanced Practice* (Brant & Wickham, 2013) (see Figure 5-1).

Motivation and Readiness to Change: Methods to Assess Readiness and Integrate Change

Motivational Interviewing

One method to determine individuals' motivation and current stage of readiness to change their behavior is through motivational interviewing (Marcus & Lewis, 2003). This type of interviewing is used with individuals who may be

Standard I. Assessment
- Use theoretical and evidence-based concepts in nursing to assess individual patient populations.
- Use appropriate evidence-based assessment techniques and instruments in collecting data, including valid and reliable instruments that assess the high-incidence problem areas (e.g., distress thermometer).

Standard II. Diagnosis
- Use evidence-based research to formulate the plan of care.

Standard III. Outcome Identification
- Ensure that expected outcomes are realistic in relation to the patient's present and potential capabilities.
- Design expected outcomes to maximize the patient's functional abilities.

Standard IV. Planning
- Include individualized physical, psychological, and social interventions in the plan of care that are
  - Supported by current evidence-based research and practice
  - Designed to achieve the stated outcomes
  - Prioritized according to the patient's needs and preferences
  - Supportive of diversity awareness

Standard V. Implementation
- Ensure that interventions are implemented in a safe, culturally competent, appropriate, caring, and humanistic manner.
- Use evidence-based research to guide implementation of interventions.

Standard VI. Evaluation
- Use evidence-based research in the evaluation of expected outcomes.

Figure 5-1. Standards Applicable to Behavior Change

Note. From *Statement on the Scope and Standards of Oncology Nursing Practice: Generalist and Advanced Practice,* by J.M. Brant and R. Wickham (Eds.), 2013, Pittsburgh, PA: Oncology Nursing Society. Copyright 2013 by Oncology Nursing Society. Adapted with permission.

ambivalent or hesitant to change (Drench, Noonan, Sharby, & Ventura, 2010). This method allows for self-examination through questioning that is flexible and patient centered, allowing individuals to discover their own barriers and plans for change (Edwards, Stapleton, Williams, & Ball, 2015). Evidence supports the efficacy of motivational interviewing in cancer survivors for lifestyle behavior changes related to exercise and physical activity (Spencer & Wheeler, 2016). Motivational interviewing has been shown to be effective both face-to-face and over the telephone, and the number of sessions may vary.

During motivational interviewing, oncology nurses can use reflective listening to help cancer survivors identify unhealthy triggers. Nurses can then create a plan to support survivors' long-term adherence to physical activity programs by summarizing and offering feedback about their responses in a nonconfrontational way (Allicock et al., 2014). The plan should be practical and individualized and should control for potential barriers while at the same time building self-efficacy (Bennett, Lyons, Winters-Stone, Nail, & Scherer, 2007). Table 5-1 outlines the components, sample questions, and rationale for each facet of motivational interviewing.

> With motivational interviewing, questions posed by oncology nurses can lead individuals to determine the choices they want to make regarding physical activity.

Internal Locus of Motivation

Through motivational interviewing, oncology nurses can assess the locus of motivation for physical activity in cancer survivors. The most powerful behavioral regulation is *intrinsic motivation*, behavior that is driven by internal rewards; many

Table 5-1. Motivational Interviewing Questions and Rationale

Objective	Sample Questions	Rationale
Setting an agenda	"Would you mind if we talked about a physical activity plan?"	Emphasizes survivor autonomy through asking permission
Exploring the survivor's desire	"Are you interested in becoming active during your day?"	Assesses the component of changing values
Exploring the survivor's ability	"Would you be able to ride your bike for 15 minutes each day?"	Assesses self-efficacy
Exploring the survivor's reasons for adding physical activity	"You said you that you are now more open to adding physical activity to your day. What makes you open to this now?"	Assesses amount of motivation
Providing information	"Did you know that physical activity has been linked to health benefits for your heart and lungs as well as a reduction in cancer recurrence (in some types of cancer)? Several options are available for an individual exercise program."	Conveys hope that options are available and that the positive effects of physical activity are related to long-term outcomes
Listening and summarizing	"What do you think of the idea of adding physical activity? It sounds like you are interested but concerned about balance. Perhaps incorporating exercises specifically for balance would be a good idea."	Summarizes personal health risks and appropriate interventions; reveals areas of ambivalence

survivors exhibit characteristics of intrinsic motivation from either prior experience with exercise, desire to maximize their health, or desire to reduce their recurrence rate for cancer (Daley & Duda, 2006). *Extrinsic motivation*, on the other hand, is behavior that is derived from external rewards or threats outside of the self. The levels of motivation in relation to physical activity and exercise are as follows:

- **Individual lacks intrinsic motivation but possesses external motivation from rewards or threats:** The individual may prefer an outline of specific goals to aid in adherence to a physical activity program and may participate in physical activity because he or she is aware of the many benefits, such as reduced risk of cancer recurrence (threat) or weight loss (reward).
- **Individual lacks or has little motivation to engage in physical activity as well as an inability to see the correlation between participation in physical activity and expected outcomes:** The individual has experienced significant fatigue, pain, or depression following too intense physical activity and may benefit from encouragement or reminders about physical activity (e.g., text messages, phone calls). The individual may do well in a group setting.
- **Individual possesses high intrinsic motivation:** The individual is able to adhere to physical activity programs more consistently and may actually require guidance on the high threshold of physical activity for his or her current health status as compared to the lower end of parameters. This individual does not need as much motivation and encouragement and may already be aware of the benefits.

The 5 A's

A model for intervention that could be integrated into a healthcare visit is the "5 A's" (see Figure 5-2) (Agency for Healthcare Research and Quality, 2008; McKinney, 2013; Vallis, 2013). This model originally was developed for clinical interventions for tobacco cessation by the National Cancer Institute as a brief intervention, requiring less than three minutes of direct patient care time. The "5 A's" also has been studied in obesity counseling, as the model revolves around behavior change theory (Vallis, 2013). The order of the different components should be altered based on the situation and patient needs.

Stages of Change

An additional framework to integrate the processes and principles of new exercise behavior for cancer survivors is the transtheoretical model of behavior change (Prochaska & Velicer, 1997). This model demonstrates that changes in health behaviors occur in stages. After determining the stage of change that the individual is experiencing, nurses can find the most appropriate and effective interventions. This provides opportunities for improving adherence to health-related activities and outcomes. Table 5-2 aligns each of the five stages of change and includes suggested strategies for promoting physical activity (Marcus & Lewis, 2003; Prochaska, Redding, & Evers, 2008).

Assess

This includes physical anthropometric measurements and exercise testing to determine current fitness level. In addition, nutrition, medications, and a full medical history should be reviewed. It is here that the nurse can determine the cancer survivor's readiness to change behavior and stage of change.

Advise

Various types of exercise can lead to improved health and promote adherence. Appropriateness of the exercise selected, realistic FITT (frequency, intensity, time, type) parameters (see Chapter 4), and self-monitoring can be reviewed.

Agree

The cancer survivor must be ready, or the conversation can be continued at a subsequent visit. If the survivor is ready, the physical activity plan can be developed.

Assist

The cancer survivor will require guidance and resources for safe physical activity and self-monitoring (e.g., target heart rate, rating of perceived exertion). The individual may require pictures of exercises if performing them at home or directions or a map to get to the group fitness location.

Arrange

Follow-up appointments to discuss the cancer survivor's performance and adherence are important. Referrals to other healthcare providers may be valuable for problem solving to reduce barriers.

Figure 5-2. The 5 A's of Integrating Behavior Change Into a Healthcare Visit

Note. Based on information from McKinney, 2013.

Table 5-2. Readiness to Change and Physical Activity Recommendation

Stage of Change	Description	Suggestions for Promoting Physical Activity and Exercise
Precontemplation	Currently inactive and not thinking about increasing physical activity	Nurse can briefly discuss the value of physical activity and exercise.
Contemplation	Inactive but is thinking about adding physical activity or exercise in the next six months	Nurse can do one or more of the following: • Share a brochure on physical activities. • Show a short video about patients being physically active. • Have patient talk with other cancer survivors about their physical activities.

(Continued on next page)

Table 5-2. Readiness to Change and Physical Activity Recommendation (Continued)

Stage of Change	Description	Suggestions for Promoting Physical Activity and Exercise
Preparation	Patient desires or is curious about physical activity and exercise in the next month; may have initiated activity but not at own individualized recommendation level	Patient can do one or more of the following: • Purchase a new pair of walking shoes or jacket. • Visit a personal trainer. • Visit a fitness center or community center. • Make plans with a friend to go for a walk or take a group fitness class. • Join a garden club. • Find a coworker to walk around the office with at lunchtime. • Ask a coworker to take a stretch break.
Action	Patient is physically active at the recommended level for less than six months	Patient has established a routine for physical activity and exercise. Patient has joined a fitness center.
Maintenance	Patient has been exercising for greater than six months at the recommended level	Physical activity and exercise are now part of patient's lifestyle.

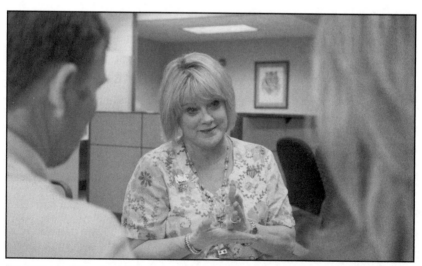

Integrate questions about behavior change and strategies to promote change into follow-up visits.

The General Self-Efficacy Scale

The General Self-Efficacy Scale can be used to assess perceived self-efficacy when the aim is to help predict coping with daily hassles that may derail an exercise program after experiencing the stress of a cancer diagnosis and associated treatment (Schwarzer & Jerusalem, 1995). This scale can be self-administered and takes about four minutes to complete; responses are scored on a four-point scale (see Figure 5-3).

The Stanford Brief Activity Survey

Physical activity surveys also can be used to assist oncology nurses. The Stanford Brief Activity Survey is one assessment that can be used to determine the amount and intensity of physical activity a person completes during the day (Taylor-Piliae et al., 2010). In this two-item survey, respondents are asked about sedentary and strenuous levels with work-related activity and intensity and frequency in leisurely activity.

The Godin-Shephard Leisure-Time Physical Activity Questionnaire

The Godin-Shephard Leisure-Time Physical Activity Questionnaire is commonly used in oncology research and behavior change. Although clear evidence for reliability and validity for this population is lacking, it was reported in a systematic review that this questionnaire may be useful for identifying determinants of leisure-time physical activity behaviors, verification of the risks or protective factors related to health-related outcomes, and evaluation of behavior change interventions on leisure-time physical activity behavior (Amireault, Godin, Lacombe,

---

1. I can always manage to solve difficult problems if I try hard enough.
2. If someone opposes me, I can find the means and ways to get what I want.
3. It is easy for me to stick to my aims and accomplish my goals.
4. I am confident that I could deal efficiently with unexpected events.
5. Thanks to my resourcefulness, I know how to handle unforeseen situations.
6. I can solve most problems if I invest the necessary effort.
7. I can remain calm when facing difficulties because I can rely on my coping abilities.
8. When I am confronted with a problem, I can usually find several solutions.
9. If I am in trouble, I can usually think of a solution.
10. I can usually handle whatever comes my way.

Scoring: 1 = Not at all true; 2 = Hardly true; 3 = Moderately true; 4 = Exactly true. Add scores for all 10 items to yield a composite score of 10–40.

Figure 5-3. The General Self-Efficacy Scale

Note. From "Generalized Self Efficacy Scale" (pp. 35–37), by R. Schwarzer and M. Jerusalem in J. Weinman, S. Wright, and M. Johnston (Eds.), *Measures in Health Psychology: A User's Portfolio. Casual and Control Beliefs*, 1995, Windsor, UK: NFER-NELSON. Copyright 1995 by NFER-NELSON. Reprinted with permission.

& Sabiston, 2015). This four-item self-administered questionnaire assesses the number of times a person engages in mild, moderate, or strenuous physical activity for at least 15 minutes during a typical week. A leisure score index is calculated and can be used to rank individuals' levels of physical activity (from low to high) and classify them as active or insufficiently active (Godin & Shephard, 1985).

Application to Oncology Nursing Practice

1. Learn more about motivational interviewing techniques. Provide patients with education materials from your oncology center (or create resources if none are available).
2. Assess cancer survivors' readiness to change based on the stages outlined in Table 5-2. Explore strategies to help cancer survivors move to the next stage.
3. Use the 5 A's (Assess, Advise, Agree, Assist, Arrange) when talking with patients or clients about physical activity and exercise.
4. Determine which method outlined in this chapter works best for your own nursing practice.
5. Seek additional education and training in behavior change through wellness coaching, which emphasizes motivational interviewing techniques that can help individuals, including cancer survivors, who are looking to improve their health.

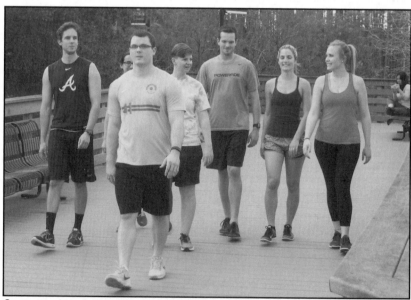

Cancer survivors in the action stage establish a routine for physical activity and exercise and are supported by walking in groups.

Summary

Each cancer survivor's readiness for physical activity and exercise is different and is an important contributing factor when creating a physical activity program. Determining motivating factors through motivational interviewing and using outcome measures can assist oncology nurses in determining the survivor's readiness to change, especially among survivors who are hesitant or ambivalent about physical activity. Promoting physical activity and exercise based on the stage of behavior change is important for creating realistic plans and maintaining long-term activity and exercise programs.

Case Study

J.R. is a 25-year-old man who was diagnosed with stage IB osteosarcoma 18 months ago. During this time, he underwent chemotherapy before and after surgery. Prior to his diagnosis, J.R. competed in 5K races and had a goal of running a half marathon (13.1 miles). He has not gone jogging since treatment began. His physical activity after his surgery has been limited to inpatient physical therapy. He is hesitant to begin jogging again because it was during training for a half marathon that his leg started hurting and he learned about his diagnosis. He does divulge that although he has been thinking about starting to run again, he does not know how to start or when would be best.

During a follow-up visit, his clinician assesses his current fitness level, advises him about exercise options, obtains mutual agreement about the plan, assists with resources, and arranges for a follow-up.

Stages of Readiness to Change	
Stage	**Actions**
Contemplation	• Share a brochure with J.R. on physical activity following major surgery and cancer diagnosis and treatment. • Talk to someone who is living with osteosarcoma and learn about their physical activity program.
Preparation	• Suggest J.R. purchase a new pair of running shoes. • Advise J.R. to visit a health clinic or physical therapy office that caters to patients with cancer. • Encourage J.R. to make plans with friends or other cancer survivors or to join a group.
Action	• J.R. has decided to find an exercise class led by a physical therapist. • He has started to trust his body again and went on his first jog.

Sample Initial Exercise Prescription				
Exercise Type	Frequency	Intensity	Time	Type
Cardiovascular	3–4 times per week	65%–75% oxygen uptake peak (VO$_2$), 11/20 on the Borg rating of perceived exertion scale	30–45 minutes with at least 5–10 minutes warm-up and cooldown with stretching	Jogging

The authors would like to acknowledge Olivia Huffman, PT, DPT, for her contribution to the case study.

References

Agency for Healthcare Research and Quality. (2008). *Clinical practice guideline: Treating tobacco use and dependence: 2008 update.* Retrieved from http://www.ahrq.gov/sites/default/files/wysiwyg/professionals/clinicians-providers/guidelines-recommendations/tobacco/clinicians/update/treating_tobacco_use08.pdf

Allicock, M., Carr, C., Johnson, L.-S., Smith, R., Lawrence, M., Kaye, L., ... Manning, M. (2014). Implementing a one-on-one peer support program for cancer survivors using a motivational interviewing approach: Results and lessons learned. *Journal of Cancer Education, 29,* 91–98. doi:10.1007/s13187-013-0552-3

Amireault, S., Godin, G., Lacombe, J., & Sabiston, C.M. (2015). The use of the Godin-Shephard Leisure-Time Physical Activity Questionnaire in oncology research: A systematic review. *BMC Medical Research Methodology, 16.* doi:10.1186/s12874-015-0045-7

Bennett, J.A., Lyons, K.S., Winters-Stone, K., Nail, L.M., & Scherer, J. (2007). Motivational interviewing to increase physical activity in long-term cancer survivors: A randomized controlled trial. *Nursing Research, 56,* 18–27. doi:10.1097/00006199-200701000-00003

Brant, J.M., & Wickham, R. (Eds.). (2013). *Statement on the scope and standards of oncology nursing practice: Generalist and advanced practice.* Pittsburgh, PA: Oncology Nursing Society.

Daley, A.J., & Duda, J.L. (2006). Self-determination, stage of readiness to change for exercise, and frequency of physical activity in young people. *European Journal of Sport Science, 6,* 231–243. doi:10.1080/17461390601012637

Drench, M., Noonan, A., Sharby, N., & Ventura, S. (2010). *Psychosocial aspects of health care* (3rd ed.). Upper Saddle River, NJ: Prentice Hall.

Edwards, E.J., Stapleton, P., Williams, K., & Ball, L. (2015). Building skills, knowledge and confidence in eating and exercise behavior change: Brief motivational interviewing training for healthcare providers. *Patient Education and Counseling, 98,* 674–676. doi:10.1016/j.pec.2015.02.006

Godin, G., & Shephard, R.J. (1985). A simple method to assess exercise behavior in the community. *Canadian Journal of Applied Sports Sciences, 10,* 141–146.

Marcus, B.H., & Lewis, B.A. (2003). Physical activity and the stages of motivational readiness for change model. *President's Council on Physical Fitness and Sports Research Digest, 4*(1), 1–8. Retrieved from https://www.presidentschallenge.org/informed/digest/docs/200303digest.pdf

McKinney, L. (2013). *Diagnosis and management of obesity.* Retrieved from http://www.aafp.org/dam/AAFP/documents/patient_care/fitness/obesity-diagnosis-management.pdf

Prochaska, J.O., Redding, C.A., & Evers, K.E. (2008). The transtheoretical model and stages of change. In K. Glanz, B.K. Rimer, & K. Viswanath (Eds.), *Health behavior and health education: Theory, research, and practice* (4th ed., pp. 97–122). San Francisco, CA: Jossey-Bass.

Prochaska, J.O., & Velicer, W.F. (1997). The transtheoretical model of health behavior change. *American Journal of Health Promotion, 12,* 38–48.

Schwarzer, R., & Jerusalem, M. (1995). Generalized self-efficacy scale. In J. Weinman, S. Wright, & M. Johnston (Eds.), *Measures in health psychology: A user's portfolio. Causal and control beliefs* (pp. 35–37). Windsor, UK: NFER-NELSON.

Spencer, J.C., & Wheeler, S.B. (2016). A systematic review of motivational interviewing interventions in cancer patients and survivors. *Patient Education and Counseling, 99,* 1099–1105. doi:10.1016/j.pec.2016.02.003

Taylor-Piliae, R.E., Fair, J.M., Haskell, W.L., Varady, A.N., Iribarren, C., Hlatky, M.A., … Fortmann, S.P. (2010). Validation of the Stanford Brief Activity Survey: Examining psychological factors and physical activity levels in older adults. *Journal of Physical Activity and Health, 7,* 87–94.

Vallis, M., Piccinini-Vallis, H., Sharma, A.M., & Freedhoff, Y. (2013). Clinical review: Modified 5 A's: Minimal intervention for obesity counseling in primary care. *Canadian Family Physician, 59,* 27–31.

CHAPTER **6**

Assessing Readiness for Physical Activity: Physical Considerations

Frances Westlake, PT, DPT, NCS, Alaina Newell, PT, DPT, WCS, CLT-LANA, and Betsy J. Becker, PT, DPT, CLT-LANA

Introduction

Daily physical activity involves movement that is performed at the individual's discretion. It is based on the frequency, intensity, time, and type of physical activity (see Chapter 4).

As a subset of physical activity, exercise is performed to improve one or more components of physical fitness: cardiovascular (aerobic) conditioning, muscular strength, muscular endurance, body composition, and flexibility. Improvement in physical fitness parameters is an outcome of exercise, and the ability to perform exercise programs safely is paramount, particularly in cancer survivors. In some cases, collaboration with a healthcare professional, such as a physical therapist, is required to ensure that the proper frequency, intensity, time, and type of exercise are provided based on individual health status. This collaboration holds true for cancer survivors throughout the cancer trajectory. This chapter reviews the process for assessing cancer survivors' physical readiness for physical activity and exercise. This chapter's content is supported in the Oncology Nursing Society's *Statement on the Scope and Standards of Oncology Nursing Practice: Generalist and Advanced Practice* (Brant & Wickham, 2013) (see Figure 6-1).

Standard I. Assessment
- Collect data from multiple sources, including the patient, the family, other care providers, and the community.

Standard II. Diagnosis
- Develop and/or validate nursing diagnoses with the patient, family, and appropriate providers, including the interdisciplinary cancer care team when possible.

Standard III. Outcome Identification
- Design expected outcomes to maximize the patient's functional abilities.
- Formulate expected outcomes in congruence with other planned therapies and recognize how planned cancer therapies influence expected outcomes.
- Ensure that expected outcomes provide direction for continuity of care.

Standard IV. Planning
- Coordinate appropriate resources and consultative services to provide continuity of care and appropriate follow-up in the plan of care.

Standard V. Implementation
- Identify community resources and support systems needed to implement the plan of care.

Standard VI. Evaluation
- Ensure that the patient, family, and members of the interdisciplinary cancer care team participate collaboratively in the evaluation process when possible.
- Communicate the patient's response with the interdisciplinary cancer care team and other agencies involved in the healthcare continuum.

Figure 6-1. Standards Applicable to Assessing Physical Readiness to Participate in Physical Activity and Exercise

Note. From *Statement on the Scope and Standards of Oncology Nursing Practice: Generalist and Advanced Practice*, by J.M. Brant and R. Wickham (Eds.), 2013, Pittsburgh, PA: Oncology Nursing Society. Copyright 2013 by Oncology Nursing Society. Adapted with permission.

Assessment for Exercise Readiness

Assess cancer survivors' health prior to designing an exercise program. The following parameters should be assessed:
- Health history
- Completion of risk assessments
- Completion of physical screening
- Relative and absolute contraindications for exercise
- Exercise testing
- Cardiovascular testing
- Submaximal cardiovascular testing

"I have always been physically active. After being diagnosed with leukemia and enduring a stem cell transplant, as well as having chronic and severe graft-versus-host disease, I am grateful that I was able to gain the mental, emotional, and physical strength to resume the physical activity that I had taken for granted."
—Ron A.

Review of Health History

An accurate review of health history is the first step in learning about individuals' capabilities in engaging in physical activity and exercise. Because of the compounding effects of cancer treatment, survivors may be at increased risk for exercise-induced events (Kenjale et al., 2014). For example, radiation poses a risk if the heart was in the treatment field and some of the patient's prior or current medications are potentially cardiotoxic. Throughout cancer survivorship, health history changes; therefore, physical activity and exercise options will change as well. Table 6-1 outlines selected health history parameters and offers specific considerations and information to be obtained prior to recommending physical activities and exercise.

Completion of Risk Assessments

The preferred method for assessing readiness to begin an exercise program is the administration of validated scales that measure an individual's risk for adverse events associated with exercise, typically cardiovascular exercise (Kenjale et al., 2014). No validated risk assessments specific to the oncology population currently exist; however, the most recognized general assessment scales are the Physical Activity Readiness Questionnaires (PAR-Q and PAR-Q+) and the American College of Sports Medicine (ACSM) exercise preparticipation screening guidelines.

PAR-Q and PAR-Q+: PAR-Q identifies cardiac risk factors that can affect participation in an exercise program (ACSM, 2014). This self-report questionnaire screens for the small number of adults for whom exercise may be inappropriate or those who should seek medical advice concerning the type of activity most suitable for them. PAR-Q+ is another tool that can be used prior to exercise participation, as it includes questions about chronic health conditions that may require further investigation by a nurse. These questionnaires are available through the Canadian Society for Exercise Physiology (see Chapter 15).

ACSM exercise preparticipation screening recommendations: ACSM recommends exercise preparticipation screening for healthy individuals who are asymptomatic (Pescatello & Riebe, 2015; Riebe et al., 2015). This screening model helps to determine the effect of exercise participation on individuals at risk for cardiovascular disease and when to consult a healthcare professional prior to participation (see Figure 6-2).

The 2015 ACSM exercise preparticipation health screening recommendations are based on three factors identified as modulators of risk for exercise-related cardiovascular events (Riebe et al., 2015):
• Current level of physical activity
• Presence of signs or symptoms or known cardiovascular, metabolic, or renal disease
• Desired intensity of exercise

Table 6-1. Health History Parameters and Cancer-Specific Considerations When Assessing for Exercise Readiness

Health History Parameter	Cancer-Specific Considerations
Current lifestyle and activity preferences	• Social versus solitary • Outdoors versus indoors • Structured versus unstructured
Health history	• Cancer history, diagnosis, progression, and treatment • Current exercise or physical activity program • Hematologic parameters • Prior experience with exercise or physical activity • Surgical procedures
Current signs and symptoms	• Anxiety, depression, or sadness • Cognitive functioning • Fatigue • Loss of balance/coordination • Neuropathy • Pain or discomfort • Sleep disturbances
Medications	• Angiotensin-converting enzyme inhibitors • Anticoagulants • Antihypertensives • Chemotherapy agents • Insulin/type 2 diabetes drugs • Statins
Presence of devices	• Bone fixators or joint replacements • Breast implants • Implanted ports • Indwelling bladder catheters • Ostomy or wound drainage bags • Peripherally inserted central catheters • Prostheses (eye, oral, limb) • Radiation implants • Testicular implants
Planned or completed oncology treatment	When the treatment will begin or was completed (days, weeks, months) and the length of the course of treatment (weeks, months) • Chemotherapy • Radiation therapy • Surgical procedure(s)

This risk assessment provides information to assess whether further exercise testing is needed to determine readiness for exercise. Cardiac testing is conducted based on a physician's prescription. Testing is conducted by an exercise physiologist, physical therapist, or physician.

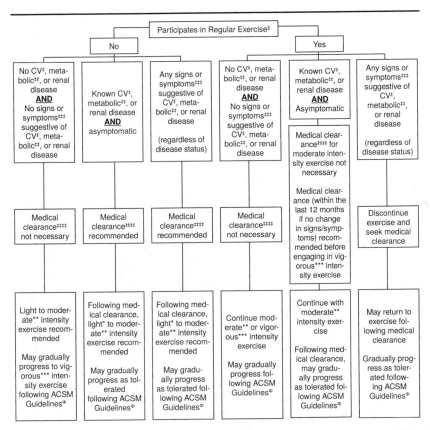

§Exercise participation, performing planned, structured physical activity at least 30 min at moderate intensity on at least 3 d wk⁻¹ for at least the last 3 months.

*Light-intensity exercise, 30% to < 40% HRR or VO_2R, 2 to < 3 METs, 9–11 RPE, an intensity that causes slight increases in HR and breathing.

**Moderate-intensity exercise, 40% to < 60% HRR or VO_2R, 3 to < 6 METs, 12–13 RPE, an intensity that causes noticeable increase in HR and breathing.

***Vigorous-intensity exercise ≥ 60% HRR or VO_2R, ≥ 6 METs, ≥ 14 RPE, an intensity that causes substantial increases in HR and breathing.

‡CVD, cardiac, peripheral vascular, or cerebrovascular disease.

‡‡Metabolic disease, type 1 and 2 diabetes mellitus.

‡‡‡Signs and symptoms, at rest or during activity; includes pain, discomfort in the chest, neck, jaw, arms, or other areas that may result from ischemia; shortness of breath at rest or with mild exertion; dizziness or syncope; orthopnea or paroxysmal nocturnal dyspnea; ankle edema; palpitations or tachycardia; intermittent claudication; known heart murmur; or unusual fatigue or shortness of breath with usual activities.

‡‡‡‡Medical clearance, approval from a health care professional to engage in exercise.

ΦACSM Guidelines, see *ACSM's Guidelines for Exercise Testing and Prescription, 9th edition,* 2014.

Figure 6-2. Exercise Preparticipation Screening Process

CV—cardiovascular; CVD—cardiovascular disease; HR—heart rate; HRR—heart rate reserve; METs—metabolic equivalent of tasks; RPE—rating of perceived exertion; VO_2R—oxygen uptake reserve

Note. From "Updating ACSM's Recommendations for Exercise Preparticipation Health Screening," by D. Riebe, B.A. Franklin, P.D. Thompson, C.E. Garber, G.P. Whitfield, M. Magal, and L.S. Pescatello, 2015, *Medicine and Science in Sports and Exercise, 47,* p. 2477. Copyright 2015 by American College of Sports Medicine. Reprinted with permission.

Completion of Physical Screening

In addition to risk assessments, physical screening using functional tests is an efficient method to gauge individuals' readiness for a general physical activity/exercise program. If performance is outside of the normal defined ranges, a referral to a physical therapist for more detailed examination and physical activity program may be warranted. These standardized tests typically are conducted by a physical therapist or exercise scientist and may include the following: five times sit to stand (5TSS), two-minute walk test (2MWT), and hand grip strength. Instructions for these three tests are presented in Figure 6-3.

Although oncology nurses may not use such testing in their oncology center, it is important to have a basic understanding of the process

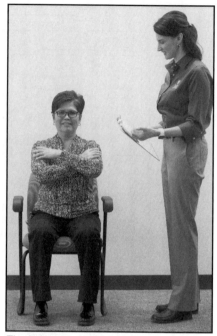

The five times sit to stand test measures functional lower limb strength.

of exercise testing. Understanding when and why the exercise tests are conducted will afford oncology nurses the opportunity to help interpret results for cancer survivors and to collaborate with the healthcare team for the selection of appropriate physical activities and exercises and programs for cancer survivors.

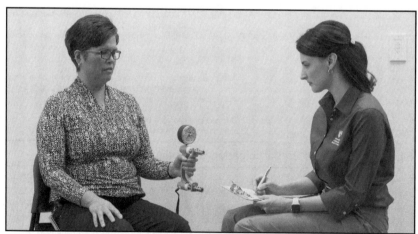

Physical therapists can test cancer survivors' hand grip strength by using a dynamometer.

Five Times Sit to Stand

Objective: Measure functional lower extremity muscle strength; could be helpful in quantifying functional change in transitional movements

Test administration:
1. Patient sits with arms folded across chest and with back against the chair. For patients who have had a stroke, it is permissible to have the impaired arm at the side or in a sling.
2. Use a standard chair with arms (keep testing chair consistent for each retest). Chair heights recorded in the literature vary (generally 43–45 cm).
3. Ensure that the chair is not secured (i.e., not against the wall or mat).

Patient instructions:
1. Instruct patient to stand fully between repetitions of the test and not to touch the back of the chair during each repetition. It is OK if the patient does touch the back of the chair, but it is not recommended.
2. Timing begins at "Go" and ends when the buttocks touch the chair after the fifth repetition.
3. Provide one practice trial before measurements are recorded. If you are concerned that the patient may fatigue with a practice trial, it is OK to demonstrate to the patient and have the patient do two repetitions to ensure he or she understands the instructions.
4. Inability to complete five repetitions without assistance or use of upper extremity support indicates failure of test. (Any modifications should be documented.)
5. Try NOT to talk to the patient during the test (may decrease patient's speed).
6. Document speed and assistance level.

Assistance levels:
- Contact guard assistance: Person requires hands-on support during test.
- Supervision: Person requires close supervision during test.
- Moderate independent: Person completes the test independently but does so with increased time or additional assistance.
- Independent: Person completes the test with normal speed and without assistance.

Time to administer: Less than five minutes

Normative data:
- Many studies report normative data for this test, including cutoff scores for when further assessment is recommended for fall risk. Several normative values are available based on health condition and age.
- The Rehabilitation Measures Database contains normative values for many of these studies and is a resource for healthcare providers to reference (www.rehabmeasures .org/Lists/RehabMeasures/DispForm.aspx?ID=1015).

Figure 6-3. Common Physical Screening Tests

(Continued on next page)

Hand Grip Strength

Objective: Measure isometric muscular strength of hand and forearm, screen for nutrition status

Equipment needed: Grip dynamometer

Test administration:
1. Person is seated in a chair with feet on the floor or foot plate of wheelchair. Knees are bent at a 90-degree angle.
2. Support the dynamometer and ensure that the participant is holding the arm being tested at a 90-degree angle (next to but not touching his/her body).

Patient instructions:
1. Squeeze the dynamometer handle twice (one practice and one test trial) with each hand while your arm is against your side and your elbow is bent at 90 degrees. The handle won't move, but the machine will show how hard you squeezed.
2. When the nurse says "squeeze," you should squeeze the handle hard (but not as hard as you can).

CLINICAL NOTE: Reduced grip strength should also be utilized when assessing a person's nutrition status. It is one of the six characteristics considered to support a diagnosis of malnutrition and benefit from medical nutrition therapy referral. Malnutrition is a major contributor to decreased functional abilities and a contributor to increased morbidity and mortality (White et al., 2012).

Normative data:
- If person falls two standard deviations below the mean, a physical therapy evaluation may be warranted.
- Many studies report normative data for grip strength related to gender, health status, and country of origin.
- The Rehabilitation Measures Database contains normative values for many of these studies and is a resource for healthcare providers to reference (www.rehabmeasures .org/Lists/RehabMeasures/DispForm.aspx?ID=1185).

Two-Minute Walk Test

Objective: Measure endurance by assessing walking distance over 2 minutes

Equipment needed: Two cones, a chair, measuring tape, and masking tape

Space needed: At least 60 feet in length

Figure 6-3. Common Physical Screening Tests

(Continued on next page)

Setup for 2-Minute Walk Test

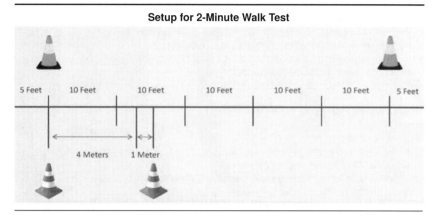

1. At 5 feet from the start, put a piece of tape 2' to 3' long across the hallway.
2. Put shorter pieces of tape at four 10-foot intervals from that piece of tape.
3. At the fifth 10-foot interval, put another piece of tape 2' to 3' long across the hallway.

Test administration:

1. Introduce the task: "This is an activity that shows how physically fit you are by seeing how far you can walk in 2 minutes. I will ask you to walk as fast as you can until I ask you to stop. I know this is hard for some people, so don't worry if you have to slow down or rest. If you do stop or slow down, start walking again as soon as you feel you are ready do so."
2. Ask the participant if there is any reason why he or she cannot do the walk. Does anything hurt or is the participant in pain? If not, have the participant walk as far as he or she can in two minutes. If the participant does not feel that he or she can do this task, note this and continue with another measure.
3. Explain to the participant that you will not talk while the participant is walking because this might affect his or her speed. You will, however, let him or her know how much time he or she has left and when he or she is almost done. One practice time is allowed.
4. Put a piece of tape on the floor to mark where the participant has stopped; the tape should be placed behind the participant's heel.
5. Direct the participant to sit down while you measure the distance from the last cone passed to the piece of tape.

Patient instructions:

1. You will start with your feet behind the line that the examiner has marked on the floor. When he or she says "Go," you will walk back and forth around the cones as fast as you can without running or hurting yourself.
2. As you pass the cone, do not stop or slow down. When the examiner tells you to stop, stop where you are on the path.

Figure 6-3. Common Physical Screening Tests

(Continued on next page)

Assistance levels:
- Contact guard assistance: Person requires hands-on support during test.
- Supervision: Person requires close supervision during test.
- Moderate independent: Person completes the test independently but does so with increased time or additional assistance.
- Independent: Person completes the test with normal speed and without assistance.

Time to administer: About 2 minutes

Normative data:
- Minimal detectable change in older adult population: 12.2 meters (40 feet) (90% confidence interval) (Connelly et al., 2009)
- Normative data for community-dwelling patients with cancer are not available.
- Mean standard deviation (Connelly et al., 2009):
  - Long-term care group: 77.5 meters (254 feet)
  - Retirement-dwelling older adults: 150.4 meters (493 feet)
- If person falls two standard deviations below the mean, a physical therapy evaluation may be warranted.
- Note deviation from a straight line during ambulation, pauses, or change in speed during the test.
- The Rehabilitation Measures Database contains additional information on normative values for many studies and is a resource for healthcare providers to reference (www.rehabmeasures.org/Lists/RehabMeasures/DispForm.aspx?ID=896).

Figure 6-3. Common Physical Screening Tests (Continued)

Note. From "NIH Toolbox for Assessment of Neurological and Behavioral Function Administrator's Manual," by National Institutes of Health, 2015. Retrieved from http://www.nihtoolbox.org/Resources/NIHToolboxiPadapp. Copyright 2015 by National Institutes of Health and Northwestern University. Adapted with permission.

Review of Absolute and Relative Contraindications for Exercise

Absolute and relative contraindications exist for those participating in cardiovascular exercise. These contraindications are applicable to all individuals, including cancer survivors. Contraindications include but are not limited to the following (Exercise and Sports Science Australia, 2011; Gibbons et al., 2002):

Absolute
- Recent significant change in the resting electrocardiogram
- Unstable angina
- Uncontrolled cardiac dysrhythmias
- Acute pulmonary embolus or pulmonary infarction

Relative
- Moderate stenotic heart disease
- Electrolyte abnormalities
- Severe arterial hypertension
- Left main coronary stenosis

Review of Cancer-Specific Conditions

Cancer-specific conditions are assessed prior to giving physical activity and exercise recommendations and include administration of chemotherapy agents, cancer site and type, chronic cancer-related conditions, and phase of cancer care.

Administration of chemotherapy: Specific chemotherapy agents can be cardiotoxic, placing survivors at risk for hypertension, arrhythmias, myocardial ischemia, and even heart failure. These toxicities can occur during treatment or develop years after completing therapy and may affect the ability of cancer survivors to participate in exercise. Anthracyclines are the most well-known chemotherapy class associated with cardiotoxicity. These agents cause a dose-dependent cardiotoxicity that is believed to be irreversible. Several other classes of chemotherapy agents also have been identified as causing cardiac toxicity, including alkylating agents, tyrosine kinase inhibitors, antimicro-tubule agents, and monoclonal antibodies. A complete chemotherapy history should be obtained from patients prior to starting any exercise program. Table 6-2 provides specific information regarding these potentially cardiotoxic agents.

Table 6-2. Common Agents Associated With Cardiotoxicity

Chemotherapy Agent	Incidence of Cardiotoxicity (%)	U.S. Food and Drug Administration–Approved Cancer Indications	Notes
Anthracyclines			Risk is dose dependent. Acute cardiotoxicity is rare. Chronic toxicity can be detected beginning the first year and up to many years after exposure.
Daunorubicin	> 10	Acute leukemia	
Doxorubicin	3–26	Breast cancer, lymphoma, sarcoma	
Epirubicin	< 1–3	Breast cancer	
Idarubicin	5–18	Acute myeloid leukemia (AML)	
Mitoxantrone	1–14	AML, prostate cancer	
Alkylating Agents			Risk is increased with high doses, older age, and previous radiation.
Cyclophospha-mide	6–28	Lymphoma, multiple myeloma, neuroblastoma, retinoblastoma	
Ifosfamide	< 1–17	Lymphoma, multiple myeloma, neuroblastoma, retinoblastoma	

(Continued on next page)

Table 6-2. Common Agents Associated With Cardiotoxicity *(Continued)*

Chemotherapy Agent	Incidence of Cardiotoxicity (%)	U.S. Food and Drug Administration–Approved Cancer Indications	Notes
Monoclonal Antibodies			
Ado-trastuzumab emtansine	1–3	HER2+ breast cancer	Increased risk with anthracyclines or paclitaxel
Bevacizumab	1–10	Glioblastoma; renal cell carcinoma; cervical, ovarian, non-small cell lung, and colorectal cancer	Increased risk with concomitant anthracyclines
Trastuzumab	2–28	HER2+ breast cancer, HER2+ gastric adenocarcinoma	Increased risk with anthracyclines or paclitaxel
Tyrosine Kinase Inhibitors			May increase risk in patients with underlying cardiac risk factors; heart failure, arrhythmias, hypertension, and thromboembolism have been reported.
Dasatinib	< 1–3.9	CML, Ph+ ALL	
Imatinib	< 1–1.7	Chronic myeloid leukemia (CML), Philadelphia chromosome–positive acute lymphoblastic leukemia (Ph+ ALL), gastrointestinal stromal tumor (GIST)	
Lapatinib	1.5–2.2	HER2+ breast cancer	
Nilotinib	2.9–15.2	CML	
Ponatinib	5	CML, Ph+ ALL	
Sunitinib	7–27	GIST, renal cell carcinoma, pancreatic neuroendocrine tumor	
Antimicrotubule Agents			Increased risk when given with anthracyclines
Docetaxel	2.3–8	Breast, prostate, head and neck, and non-small cell lung cancer; gastric adenocarcinoma	

(Continued on next page)

Table 6-2. Common Agents Associated With Cardiotoxicity *(Continued)*

Chemotherapy Agent	Incidence of Cardiotoxicity (%)	U.S. Food and Drug Administration– Approved Cancer Indications	Notes
Paclitaxel	1–2	Ovarian, breast, and small cell lung cancer; Kaposi sarcoma	
Proteasome Inhibitors			Increased risk with older adult patients
Bortezomib	5–8	Multiple myeloma, lymphoma	
Carfilzomib	6–8	Multiple myeloma	

Note. Based on information from Ariad Pharmaceuticals Inc., 2015; Bristol-Myers Squibb, 2015; Genentech, Inc., 2015; Novartis Pharmaceuticals Corporation, 2015; Onyx Pharmaceuticals, 2016; Pfizer Inc., 2015; Schimmel et al., 2004; Shah & Nohria, 2015; Truong et al., 2014; WG Critical Care, LLC, 2015; Yu et al., 2014.

Cancer site and type: Specific cancer sites and types (e.g., breast, colon, head and neck, lung, prostate) have their own considerations that oncology nurses should acknowledge when recommending physical activity and exercise. These conditions and recommendations are presented in Chapter 7.

Chronic cancer-related conditions: Physical activity and exercise recommendations for specific cancer-related chronic considerations, such as lymphedema, cachexia, and bone loss, are presented in Chapter 12.

Phase of cancer care: Physical activity and exercise recommendations are modified throughout the cancer trajectory. Chapter 13 discusses physical activity and exercise related to metastatic disease and end-of-life care.

Review of Hematologic Parameters

In addition to physical assessment parameters, hematologic parameters should be reviewed to ensure safe and appropriate physical activities and exercise. Blood laboratory values for the oncology population—especially for those receiving chemotherapy or bone marrow transplantation or undergoing inpatient treatment—must be considered when planning exercise programs. This information should be reviewed prior to initiating physical activity or an exercise program by both cancer survivors and the oncology team. Individuals should be taught to self-monitor for signs of bruising or bleeding before, during, and after exercising.

In addition, low hematocrit and hemoglobin levels due to chemotherapy treatments may result in impaired oxygen delivery to exercising tissues (e.g., muscles, myocardium). This impaired oxygen delivery may result in dizziness, fatigue, leg cramping, shortness of breath, rapid heart rate (compensatory tachycardia), low oxygen saturation, gait disturbance, tingling and numbness, exercise intolerance, and high rating of perceived exertion (RPE) on the Borg scale (see Chapter 4). Exercises and physical activities based on hematocrit and hemoglobin counts as well as guidelines for exercise based on platelet counts are available at the University of Pittsburgh Medical Center's website (www.upmc.com/patients-visitors/education).

Exercise Testing

Exercise testing is a battery of tests administered by exercise physiologists, physical therapists, and physician specialists to determine individuals' ability to participate in moderate- and high-intensity activities or exercises. It is recommended that routine exercise testing is performed only with individuals who are planning to exercise at a vigorous intensity (ACSM, 2014; Riebe et al., 2015). However, individuals may be referred to their healthcare professional for clearance to engage in exercise based on clinical judgment and decision making by following the preparticipation screening process shown in Figure 6-2.

Currently, the National Comprehensive Cancer Network® and ACSM do not specifically list recommendations regarding exercise testing in cancer survivors prior to engaging in exercise. Each oncology center should have its own process for determining physical readiness for exercise in cancer survivors. For centers looking for guidance to establish processes or protocols for exercise testing, the information in this chapter can serve as a guide.

Cardiovascular Testing

Maximal and submaximal cardiovascular testing are the two types of exercise testing.

Maximal cardiovascular testing: This testing requires participants to exercise to the point of volitional fatigue and requires medical supervision and emergency equipment. It uses open circuit spirometry to allow for accurate measurement of maximal oxygen uptake (VO_2 max) and anaerobic threshold (ACSM, 2014). Although some cancer survivors may be candidates for maximal cardiovascular testing, the majority of individuals are better suited to undergo submaximal cardiovascular testing.

Submaximal cardiovascular testing: This testing allows for VO_2 max to be estimated from established data. The test is stopped when the individuals achieve a predetermined submaximal exertional level. Submaximal cardiovascular testing usually has a predetermined endpoint that is either symptom limited or determined when patients reach 85% of their maximum heart rate (MHR).

Two common submaximal cardiovascular tests are the modified Bruce protocol and the six-minute walk test (6MWT) (Schmidt, Vogt, Thiel, Jäger, &

Banzer, 2013; Schmitz et al., 2010). The 6MWT, like the 2MWT, does not require a treadmill and does not have a predetermined endpoint of MHR. This test would be a preferred option for low- to moderate-functioning cancer survivors.

The ACSM (2014) guidelines recommend that patients at cardiovascular risk monitor their heart rate, blood pressure, RPE, dyspnea (shortness of breath), oxygen saturation, pain levels, and presence of angina before, during, and after each session to ensure safe physical activity and exercise.

The modified Bruce protocol was initially developed to diagnose coronary heart disease. The protocol is now used in a variety of patient populations, including the oncology population, as a submaximal cardiovascular assessment (Noonan & Dean, 2000). Patients walk on a treadmill at 1.7 miles per hour at 0% grade (zero stage), 5% (one-half-stage), or 10% (Noonan & Dean, 2000). Their heart rate, blood pressure, oxygen saturation, pain level, presence of angina, and RPE should be determined prior to starting the program. At each stage and following the test, these measures should again be assessed.

The testing is stopped when patients either reach 85% of the predicted MHR for their age or demonstrate symptoms outlined above. In order for a stage to be considered completed, patients must complete the full duration (three minutes) of the test (Noonan & Dean, 2000). MHR can be estimated by one of the following methods: $220 - \text{age}$ or $206.9 - (0.67 \times \text{age})$ (ACSM, 2014).

Important exercise planning and training effectiveness can be gained by performing the modified Bruce protocol at evaluation and scheduled intervals. It provides information on the stage the patient completed, exercise duration (minutes and seconds), HR, RPE, and dyspnea at each stage. Patients' aerobic capacity, based on age and gender, can be determined from their peak VO_2. Patients' estimated peak VO_2 max is determined from the following calculations:

• T = Total time measured in minutes and fractions of a minute (e.g., a test time of 9 minutes 30 seconds would be written as T = 9.5)
• Women (active or sedentary): peak VO_2 (ml/kg/min) = $4.38(T) - 3.90$
• Men (active or sedentary): peak VO_2 (ml/kg/min) = $2.94(T) + 7.65$

If it is determined that the modified Bruce protocol is unsafe or too aggressive, or if the patient is uncomfortable or unable to walk on a treadmill, performing the 6MWT may be more appropriate. This test can be used as an alternative to submaximal treadmill testing to gauge patients' aerobic capacity and tolerance to physical activity. The 6MWT routinely is used in healthy older adults and cardiac and pulmonary patients and has been minimally studied in the oncology population. It has been demonstrated to be equally valid and reliable for patients with cancer, but age and gender norms have not been established for this population (Schmidt et al., 2013).

Table 6-3 includes the mean distance (in feet) for community-dwelling older adults (by age and gender) for the 6MWT and can be useful for reference when assessing the cancer survivor's results (Steffen, Hacker, & Mollinger, 2002).

Table 6-3. Six-Minute Walk Test* Mean Distance in Feet by Age and Gender (Community-Dwelling Older Adults)

Age (years)	Distance in Feet—Male	Distance in Feet—Female
60–69	1876.64	1765.09
70–79	1729.00	1545.28
80–89	1368.11	1286.09

*This testing should be performed by a healthcare professional experienced with the protocols and who has the necessary equipment to accurately assess the patient.

Note. Based on information from Steffen et al., 2002.

Application to Oncology Nursing Practice

1. Collaborate with your oncology team to establish your oncology center's protocol for exercise risk assessment. Learn when exercise screening and testing is recommended, where it is performed, and how the results are interpreted. Develop or compare your oncology center's protocols against those described in this chapter.
2. Review the risk assessments and determine if your oncology center uses these or other assessments. Talk with your oncology team to determine if these assessments would be applicable for your patient population.
3. Review the cardiovascular testing and physical screening measures (5TSS, 2MWT, hand grip strength). Determine if your oncology center uses these or other measures. Talk with your oncology team to determine if these measurements would be applicable for your patient population.
4. Review the relative and absolute contraindications for exercise. Compare these contraindications with those used by your oncology center.
5. Review the cancer-specific functional considerations in Chapter 7.

Summary

Being physically active is safe for most people, including cancer survivors throughout their cancer care. Exercise is a subset of physical activity and requires additional assessment to ensure safety in individuals undergoing or completing cancer treatment. This readiness for exercise can be assessed by oncology nurses and oncology team members using standard measures and a common-sense approach.

Case Study

G.W. is a 70-year-old woman with stage III breast cancer. Currently, she uses a compression garment for lymphedema on her right arm. G.W. played cards twice a week and participated in water aerobics once a week before her cancer diagnosis. She lives with her husband and two cats in a ranch-style home. G.W. expresses feeling "wiped out" by the time she gets from the parking lot to her card club. Her goal is to start exercising again. She has increased knee pain due to her osteoarthritis. Certain contraindications must be taken into consideration about G.W. (see Figure 6-4).

Relevant Laboratory Values
- Hemoglobin: 8.2 g/dl
- Platelet count: 53 × 10^9/L

Medical History
- Osteopenia
- Knee osteoarthritis

Medications
Completed chemotherapy of doxorubicin (anthracycline) treatment about one month ago and currently is taking an aromatase inhibitor.

Absolute Contraindications
- Hemoglobin below 8 g/dl
- Active infection
- Excessive pain
- No heat in involved quadrant

Relative Contraindications
- Hemoglobin 8–10 g/dl: light exercise until levels rise above 10 g/dl
- Public gyms to be avoided while on immunosuppressant medication if white blood cell values are below 500/mm^3
- Rapid exacerbation of lymphedema
- Unmanaged lymphedema
- New redness in the involved extremity as it may be a sign of infection
- Temperature greater than 100°F (37.78°C)
- Neutrophil count less than or equal to 0.5 × 10^9
- History of doxorubicin (anthracycline) chemotherapy

Figure 6-4. Contraindications to Exercise for G.W.

Using the American College of Sports Medicine exercise preparticipation health screening guidelines, the assessment for G.W. is as follows:
- Participates in regular exercise: No
- Known cardiovascular or metabolic disease: No
- Signs and symptoms of cardiovascular or metabolic disease: No
- Interpretation: Medical clearance not necessary. Light- to moderate-intensity exercise is recommended.

Target Heart Rate Calculation

• Determine target training heart rate (HR) using Karvonen formula:
   – Maximum HR (MHR) = 220 (constant) – 70 (patient's age) = 150 beats per minute (bpm)
   – HR reserve = 150 (MHR) – 73 (resting HR [RHR]) = 77 bpm
 • Initial desired exercise intensity = light to moderate (30%–50% MHR) (96–112 bpm)
   – Target training HR = 77 (HR reserve) × 0.5 (desired intensity) + 73 (RHR) = 112 bpm
   – Target training HR = 77 (HR reserve) × 0.3 (desired intensity) + 73 (RHR) = 96 bpm

Sample Initial Exercise Prescription				
Exercise Type	Frequency	Intensity	Time	Type
Strength	2–3 times per week	10–15 reps maximum	Working 8–10 major muscle groups	Free weights, machines, body weight, or resistance bands
Cardiovascular	5–7 days per week	Light to start (up to 50% maximum heart rate or rating of perceived exertion of 2–3/10 Individual should be able to easily talk during exercise without feeling out of breath.	3 or 4 10-minute intervals that total 30–40 minutes per session	Walking indoors or outdoors; return to water aerobics when ready
Flexibility	2–7 times per week	To the point of gentle resistance (low load)	3 times per day for 30-second holds	Prolonged stretching to large muscle groups

The authors would like to acknowledge Susanne Liewer, PharmD, BCOP, for her contribution to this chapter, Sara Bills, PT, DPT, GCS, for her critical analysis and important feedback, and Olivia Huffman, PT, DPT, Kara Tischer, PT, DPT, and Kelly McCormick, PT, DPT, for their contributions to the case study.

References

American College of Sports Medicine. (2014). *ACSM's guidelines for exercise testing and prescription* (9th ed.). Philadelphia, PA: Wolters Kluwer Health/Lippincott Williams & Wilkins.

Ariad Pharmaceuticals Inc. (2015). *Iclusig® (ponatinib)* [Package insert]. Cambridge, MA: Author.

Brant, J.M., & Wickham, R. (Eds.). (2013). *Statement on the scope and standards of oncology nursing practice: Generalist and advanced practice.* Pittsburgh, PA: Oncology Nursing Society.

Bristol-Myers Squibb. (2015). *Sprycel® (dasatinib)* [Package insert]. Princeton, NJ: Author.

Connelly, D.M., Thomas, B.K., Cliffe, S.J., Perry, W.M., & Smith, R.E. (2009). Clinical utility of the 2-minute walk test for older adults living in long-term care. *Physiotherapy Canada, 61,* 78–87. doi:10.3138/physio.61.2.78

Exercise and Sports Science Australia. (2011). Contraindications for physical activity/exercise. Retrieved from http://exerciseismedicine.org.au/wp-content/uploads/2011/07/contraindica tions-for-physical-activity-and-exercise-v1.0.pdf

Genentech, Inc. (2015). *Kadcyla® (ado-trastuzumab emtansine)* [Package insert]. South San Francisco, CA: Author.

Gibbons, R.J., Balady, G.J., Bricker, J.T., Chaitman, B.R., Fletcher, G.F., Froelicher, V.F., … Smith, S.C., Jr. (2002). ACC/AHA 2002 guideline update for exercise testing: Summary article. *Journal of the American College of Cardiology, 40,* 1531–1540.

Kenjale, A.A., Hornsby, W.E., Crowgey, T., Thomas, S., Herndon, J.E., II, Khouri, M.G., … Jones, L.W. (2014). Pre-exercise participation cardiovascular screening in a heterogeneous cohort of adult cancer patients. *Oncologist, 19,* 999–1005. doi:10.1634/theoncologist.2014-0078

Noonan, V., & Dean, E. (2000). Submaximal exercise testing: Clinical application and interpretation. *Physical Therapy, 80,* 782–807.

Novartis Pharmaceuticals Corporation. (2015). *Tasigna® (nilotinib)* [Package insert]. East Hanover, NJ: Author.

Onyx Pharmaceuticals. (2016). *Kyprolis® (carfilzomib)* [Package insert]. Thousand Oaks, CA: Author.

Pescatello, L.S., & Riebe, D. (2015). ACSM scientific roundtable: Updating recommendations for exercise preparticipation health screening. Retrieved from https://www.acsm. org/docs/default-source/publications/neacsm-2015-presentation-preparticipation-health -screeningEC3E1A47FA08.pdf?sfvrsn=0

Pfizer Inc. (2015). *Sutent® (sunitinib malate)* [Package insert]. New York, NY: Author.

Riebe, D., Franklin, B.A., Thompson, P.D., Garber, C.E., Whitfield, G.P., Magal, M., & Pescatello, L.S. (2015). Updating ACSM's recommendations for exercise preparticipation health screening. *Medicine and Science in Sports and Exercise, 47,* 2473–2479. doi:10.1249/ MSS.0000000000000664

Schimmel, K.J., Richel, D.J., van den Brink, R.B., & Guchelaar, H.J. (2004). Cardiotoxicity of cytotoxic drugs. *Cancer Treatment Reviews, 30,* 181–191. doi:10.1016/j.ctrv.2003.07.003

Schmidt, K., Vogt, L., Thiel, C., Jäger, E., & Banzer, W. (2013). Validity of the six-minute walk test in cancer patients. *International Journal of Sports Medicine, 34,* 631–636. doi:10.1055/s-0032-1323746

Schmitz, K.H., Courneya, K.S., Matthews, C., Demark-Wahnefried, W., Galvão, D.A., Pinto, B.M., … Schwartz, A.L. (2010). American College of Sports Medicine roundtable on exercise guidelines for cancer survivors. *Medicine and Science in Sports and Exercise, 42,* 1409–1426. doi:10.1249/MSS.0b013e3181e0c112

Shah, S., & Nohria A. (2015). Advanced heart failure due to cancer therapy. *Current Cardiology Reports, 17*(4), 16. doi:10.1007/s11886-015-0570-3

Steffen, T.M., Hacker, T.A., & Mollinger, L. (2002). Age- and gender-related test performance in community-dwelling elderly people: Six-Minute Walk Test, Berg Balance Scale, Timed Up and Go Test, and gait speeds. *Physical Therapy, 82,* 128–137.

Truong, J., Yan, A.T., Cramarossa, G., & Chan, K.K. (2014). Chemotherapy-induced cardiotoxicity: Detection, prevention, and management. *Canadian Journal of Cardiology, 30,* 869–878. doi:10.1016/j.cjca.2014.04.029

WG Critical Care, LLC. (2015). *Paclitaxel injection* [Package insert]. Paramus, NJ: Author.

White, J.V., Guenter, P., Jensen, G., Malone, A., & Schofield, M. (2012). Consensus statement of the Academy of Nutrition and Dietetics/American Society for Parenteral and Enteral Nutrition: Characteristics recommended for the identification and documentation of adult malnutrition (undernutrition). *Journal of the Academy of Nutrition and Dietetics, 112,* 730–738. doi:10.1016/j.jand.2012.03.012

Yu, A.F., Steingart, R.M., & Fuster, V. (2014). Cardiomyopathy associated with cancer therapy. *Journal of Cardiac Failure, 20,* 841–852. doi:10.1016/j.cardfail.2014.08.004

CHAPTER 7

Evaluating Tolerance and Adherence to Physical Activity

Frances Westlake, PT, DPT, NCS, Alaina Newell, PT, DPT, WCS, CLT-LANA, and Betsy J. Becker, PT, DPT, CLT-LANA

Introduction

Once psychosocial and physical readiness (e.g., health history, cardiovascular risk, strength, flexibility) have been assessed, a physical activity and exercise program can be created for the cancer survivor. Using the FITT principle (see Chapter 4), oncology nurses collaborate with cancer survivors and healthcare team members to determine the physical activities and exercises that are achievable. Over time, the team evaluates these programs for adherence and outcomes. This chapter synthesizes the FITT principle with current guidelines, providing a process to create physical activity and exercise programs for survivors. Evaluation parameters are presented to measure health-related outcomes. This chapter's content is supported in the Oncology Nursing Society's *Statement on the Scope and Standards of Oncology Nursing Practice: Generalist and Advanced Practice* (Brant & Wickham, 2013) (see Figure 7-1).

Creating Physical Activity and Exercise Programs

Because physical activity and exercise play a vital role in cancer prevention and cancer survivorship (see Chapter 2), participation in a regular program of

Standard I. Assessment

- Collect data in the following high-incidence problem areas. These areas may include but are not limited to the following:
  - Mobility
    * Past and present level of mobility and overall function
    * Risk for decreased mobility
    * Impact of fatigue on mobility
    * Complications related to decreased mobility
  - Survivorship: Patient/family understanding of the need for adherence to long-term follow-up

Standard II. Diagnosis

- Use evidence-based research to formulate the plan of care.

Standard III. Outcome Identification

- Develop expected outcomes collaboratively with the patient, family, interdisciplinary cancer care team, and other providers when possible.
- Ensure that expected outcomes are realistic in relation to the patient's present and potential capabilities.
- Design expected outcomes to maximize the patient's functional abilities.
- Formulate expected outcomes in congruence with other planned therapies and recognize how planned cancer therapies influence expected outcomes.
- Ensure that expected outcomes provide direction for continuity of care.
- Assign a realistic time period for expected outcomes for achievement or reevaluation and be aware of the timing of side effects and normal physiologic events associated with cancer treatment and align expected outcomes accordingly.
- Develop expected outcomes for each of the high-incidence problem areas at a level consistent with the patient's physical, psychological, social, and spiritual capacities, cultural background, and value system. The expected outcomes include but are not limited to the following:
  - Mobility: The patient and/or family
    * Explain the relationship between fatigue and exercise balance.
    * Describe an appropriate management plan to integrate alteration in mobility into lifestyle.
    * Describe optimal levels of activities of daily living at a level consistent with disease state and treatment.
  - Survivorship: The patient and/or family
    * Participate in long-term follow-up at appropriate intervals as identified in the survivorship plan.

Standard IV. Planning

- Include individualized physical, psychological, and social interventions in the plan of care that are
  - Supported by current evidence-based research and practice
  - Designed to achieve the stated outcomes
  - Prioritized according to the patient's needs and preferences
  - Supportive of diversity awareness

Figure 7-1. Standards Applicable to Physical Activity and Exercise Tolerance and Adherence

(Continued on next page)

Standard V. Implementation
• Use evidence-based research to guide implementation of interventions.

Standard VI. Evaluation
• Maintain a systematic and ongoing evaluation process.
• Collect evaluation data from all pertinent sources.
• Compare actual findings to expected findings.
• Use evidence-based research in the evaluation of expected outcomes.

Figure 7-1. Standards Applicable to Physical Activity and Exercise Tolerance and Adherence *(Continued)*

Note. From *Statement on the Scope and Standards of Oncology Nursing Practice: Generalist and Advanced Practice,* by J.M. Brant and R. Wickham (Eds.), 2013, Pittsburgh, PA: Oncology Nursing Society. Copyright 2013 by Oncology Nursing Society. Adapted with permission.

physical activity and exercise is important (Stevinson, Lawlor, & Fox, 2004). When creating a physical activity and exercise program, the oncology nurse engages the survivor in the creation process by doing the following:
• Learning the types of exercise or physical activity the survivor enjoys
• Assessing the current FITT principle: What is the individual's current frequency of activities, intensity (i.e., low, moderate, vigorous), amount of time spent in activities, and the type of activities performed?
• Shaping a program that will vary throughout oncology treatments
• Teaching ways to assess and self-monitor cardiovascular, muscular conditioning, and flexibility during and after activity.

A well-rounded physical activity and exercise program integrates a variety of exercises, including aspects of cardiovascular (aerobic) exercise and strength and flexibility training (see Chapter 4). The American College of Sports Medicine (ACSM) has provided guidelines for a well-rounded exercise program in any population, including the oncology population (ACSM, 2014; Schmitz et al., 2010). General recommendations for cardiovascular, muscular strength and endurance, and flexibility exercise are outlined in Figure 7-2. Modifications for special oncology populations, such as cancer survivors with lymphedema and bone metastases, are described in Chapters 12 and 13.

Evaluating Physical Activity and Exercise Programs

Successful physical activity and exercise programs include two components: exercise tolerance and exercise adherence. Both of these components change during and after cancer treatment. The survivor's tolerance of and adherence to the physical activity and exercise program are evaluated at every office or clinic

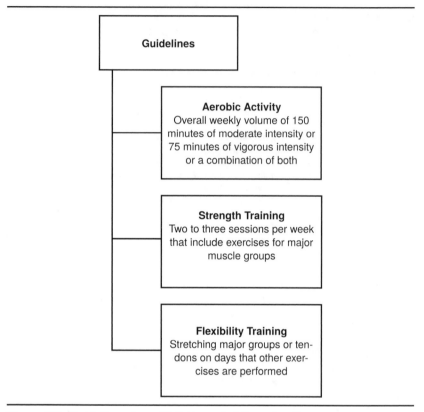

Figure 7-2. Guidelines for a Well-Rounded Exercise Program

visit. Between office visits, oncology nurses can follow up with the cancer survivor at least once a week either in person or by phone, email, or telemedicine. For those who have completed oncology treatment, follow-up is recommended based on individual needs and determined by both the healthcare team and the survivor.

Application to Oncology Nursing Practice: Evaluating Exercise Tolerance

1. Teach cancer survivors the signs and symptoms that indicate when they need to stop their session of exercise or physical activity (ACSM, 2014).
   • Onset of chest pain

- Increasing nervous system symptoms (e.g., ataxia, dizziness, confusion, nausea)
- Signs of poor perfusion (e.g., cyanosis, pallor)
- Shortness of breath, excessive fatigue, wheezing, leg cramps
- Failure of heart rate to increase with increased exertion
- Subjective feeling (e.g., "I just don't feel right/good.")
- Exercising beyond the prescribed intensity (e.g., above target heart rate or rating of perceived exertion [RPE])

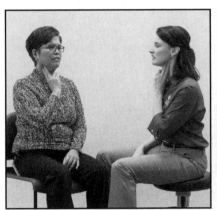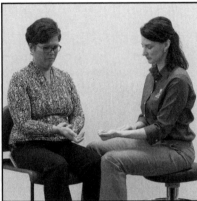

Teaching cancer survivors how to measure their carotid (left) or radial (right) pulse can help them determine the desired exercise intensity.

2. Teach cancer survivors how to measure their radial and carotid pulses to determine the desired exercise intensity (target heart rate range).
3. Teach cancer survivors how to calculate and measure their target training heart rate during exercise by using the Karvonen formula:

Maximum HR (MHR) = 220 (constant) − (age) = _____ beats per minute (bpm)

HR reserve = (MHR) − (Resting HR) = ____ bpm

Initial desired exercise intensity range = Light to moderate (40%–50% of target HR)

40% Target training HR = (HR reserve) × 0.4 (desired intensity) + (RHR) = $\underline{X}$ bpm

50% Target training HR = (HR reserve) × 0.5 (desired intensity) + (RHR) = $\underline{Y}$ bpm

Range = X–Y bpm

4. Teach cancer survivors how to measure their RPE. RPE (see Chapters 4 and 6) is a reliable scale for individuals to determine their perceived effort in addition to strain, discomfort, or fatigue that they experience during physical activity. RPE is a psychophysiologic scale that allows individuals to rate their own perception of effort by using their mind and body versus physiologic symptoms only. Studies have shown that this scale has a linear relationship with heart rate and oxygen uptake (ACSM, 2014). This feature allows the scale to be used during exercise, especially when cancer survivors demonstrate a blunted or difficult heart rate response, such as when on beta-blocker medication. Individuals must view the scale when rating their exertion for a reliable measurement (see Chapter 4).

5. Evaluate cancer survivors' tolerance to the established physical activity program, as the program progresses in frequency, intensity, and/or time (duration). Ongoing communication with cancer survivors is crucial to ensure their tolerance of the established program and to determine if changes to the program are needed. Evaluation topics to discuss are as follows:
    • Changes in health: Consider cardiac retesting or consultation with physical or occupational therapists if new cardiovascular or musculoskeletal issues arise.
    • Changes in treatment protocol: The addition of chemotherapy, radiation therapy, or surgery can affect tolerance to physical activity.
    • Adherence to FITT-based activity or exercise program: Assess the reasons why the cancer survivor may not be adherent; use motivational interviewing techniques (see Chapter 5).
    • Inclusion of aerobic, conditioning, and flexibility activities and exercises: Ensure that the physical activity and exercise program is balanced in relation to the current cancer treatment plan to avoid fatigue or other symptoms.
    • Need to change the FITT-based activity or exercise program: Over time, the cancer survivor's body will adapt to the activity or exercise program, and the program will need to be changed (i.e., principle of adaptation). The change may be an increase in frequency, intensity, time, or type of activity or exercise.

Application to Oncology Nursing Practice: Exercise Adherence

1. Educate yourself about physical activity and exercise programming. Health professionals educated about exercise may reduce barriers to physical activity and exercise participation (Blaney, Lowe-Strong,

Rankin-Watt, Campbell, & Gracey, 2013; National Comprehensive Cancer Network®, 2016). Adhering to an exercise program is difficult for the general population, regardless of a cancer diagnosis, due to lack of time, lack of motivation, and difficulty of knowing how to modify if symptoms appear.

2. Teach cancer survivors and their families how to track their physical activity and exercise daily and weekly. Tracking may help with exercise adherence and can be completed simply with a handwritten log or an online tracking program. With the increased accessibility and lower costs of mHealth applications (e.g., wearable physical activity monitors and mobile apps), automatic reminders and group sharing of exercise minutes may assist with adherence (Cadmus-Bertram, Marcus, Patterson, Parker, & Morey, 2015).

3. Teach cancer survivors and their families about the benefits of group exercise, including group support and accountability. Groups may be informally created among cancer survivors themselves or more formally through a community gym, medically based fitness center, or medical center. Van Gerpen and Becker (2013) reported the outcomes for an evidence-based cancer recovery program in a community that included biweekly small group exercise and education on a variety of topics once per week. This translation of evidence to practice showed participant improvements that were independent of cancer type, extent of disease, or treatment status. Exercise sessions were individualized but completed in a supervised group setting that was led by a physical therapist or exercise specialist.

Summary

Creating and evaluating physical activity programs for cancer survivors, as well as for oneself, is not an easy task. Physical activity programs for cancer survivors should include aerobic, strength training, and flexibility components. Special considerations of different cancer types should be considered (see Table 7-1). Exercise tolerance can be measured by individuals using the target heart rate and RPE to ensure the achievement of appropriate exercise intensity. Adhering to a physical activity program can be a challenge, and oncology nurses are prepared for that challenge by integrating cancer survivors' psychosocial readiness to change and physical readiness for activity and exercise with the FITT principle. Teaching cancer survivors how to measure their own physical activity and exercise outcomes, such as physical changes (e.g., heart rate, RPE), activity tolerance, and adherence, will help survivors maintain and improve their physical activity awareness. Involving family members in physical activity and exercise programs is a means of promoting health and companionship.

Table 7-1. Exercise Recommendations and Considerations Based on Cancer Type

Type	Pre-Exercise Assessment	Aerobic Exercise Training	Resistance Training	Flexibility Training
Breast cancer	Evaluate arm and shoulder mobility prior to upper body exercise (including girth to screen for lymphedema). 1–10 rep maximum can be safely demonstrated for individuals at risk for lymphedema.	Same as age-appropriate guidelines Be aware of fracture risk.	Start with a supervised program. No upper limit to which survivors can progress	Same as age-appropriate guidelines
Prostate cancer	Evaluate muscle strength and wasting before exercise.	Same as age-appropriate guidelines Be aware of fracture risk.	Add pelvic floor exercises for those who undergo radical prostatectomy.	Same as age-appropriate guidelines
Colorectal cancer	Evaluate established infection prevention behaviors for patients with an ostomy before engaging in exercise training more vigorous than a walking program.	Same as age-appropriate guidelines Physician permission is recommended for patients with an ostomy before participating in contact sports.	For patients with a stoma, start with low resistance and progress resistance slowly. Consider pelvic floor weakness. Referral to a physical therapist may be warranted.	Avoid increasing intra-abdominal pressure for patients with an ostomy.
Adult hematologic (hematopoietic stem cell transplantation [HSCT])	No specific medical assessments are recommended prior to starting an exercise program. Take *current* laboratory values into consideration.	OK to exercise every day. Lighter intensity and lower progression of intensity is recommended. Avoid overtraining, given immune effects of vigorous exercise.	May be more important than aerobic exercise in bone marrow transplant patients	Same as age-appropriate guidelines

(Continued on next page)

Table 7-1. Exercise Recommendations and Considerations Based on Cancer Type *(Continued)*

Type	Pre-Exercise Assessment	Aerobic Exercise Training	Resistance Training	Flexibility Training
Adult hematologic (non-HSCT)	No specific medical assessments are recommended before starting an exercise program. Take *current* laboratory values into consideration.	Same as age-appropriate guidelines	Same as age-appropriate guidelines	Same as age-appropriate guidelines
Gynecologic cancer	Evaluate lower extremity lymphedema before vigorous aerobic or resistance training.	Same as age-appropriate guidelines	Same as age-appropriate guidelines No data on the safety of resistance training in women with lower extremity lymphedema Proceed with caution if patient has had lymph node removal and/or undergone radiation. Consider pelvic floor impairments such as weakness, high tone, pain, and incontinence. Referral to physical therapist may be warranted.	Same as age-appropriate guidelines

Note. Based on information from Schmitz et al., 2010.

Case Study

B.L. is a 46-year-old woman who was recently diagnosed with stage II breast cancer. She was treated with surgical mastectomy and reconstruction. She recently finished eight chemotherapy treatments; no radiation is planned at this time. B.L. reports to her oncology nurse that she would like to start running again. She has one adult child and was an avid runner prior to beginning treatment. She does not currently work but enjoys gardening and hosting parties for her group of friends.

B.L. completed a modified Bruce protocol in 4 minutes, 9 seconds. Her estimated peak VO$_2$ was 14.28 ml/kg/min, which classifies her as "very poor" fitness status. She is limited in the bilateral shoulder flexion range of motion and has been educated on lymphedema risk reduction. Recommendation for this patient is to take advantage of specialized community classes for cancer survivors in which fitness instructors will keep in mind contraindications and precautions (see Figure 7-3).

Height/weight	• Height: 5'4" • Weight: 120 lbs • BMI: 21 • Healthy weight
Vitals	• Blood pressure: 118/74 mm Hg • Resting heart rate: 68 bpm • Respiratory rate: 16 breaths per minute • Temperature: 98.6°F (37°C)
Assessment	• Five times sit to stand test: 8 seconds (normal) • Hand grip strength test: 46 kg right; 46 kg left (normal)

Figure 7-3. Additional Patient Information

BMI—body mass index; bpm—beats per minute

Sample Initial Exercise Prescription				
Exercise Type	Frequency	Intensity	Time	Type
Strength training	1–2 times per week	One set, 8–10 reps to start, with light weights For upper extremity exercises, the individual would progress by the smallest increments after completing 2–3 sessions with the same weights and sets.	8–10 exercises addressing major muscle groups	Weight lifting under trainer supervision

(Continued on next page)

Sample Initial Exercise Prescription *(Continued)*				
Exercise Type	Frequency	Intensity	Time	Type
Cardio-vascular	3–5 times per week, increas-ing short periods of activity daily	Light to start (up to 50% maximum heart rate or rat-ing of perceived exertion [RPE] of 2–3/10) Individual should be able to easily talk during exercise without feeling out of breath (see Table 4-3 in Chap-ter 4).	Intervals of 5 minutes active, 5 minutes rest Progress to 8–10 con-tinuous minutes 1–3 bouts/day.	Walking on the tread-mill
Flexibility	2–3 times per week	Low load to point of resistance while maintaining proper position	10–15 min-utes	Yoga
Sample Moderate Exercise Progression				
Cardio-vascular	3–5 times per week	Moderate physical exertion (50%–70% maximum heart rate or RPE of 4/10)	10 minutes active, 5 minutes rest Progress to 15–25 continu-ous min-utes, 1–3 bouts/day.	Jogging or powerwalk-ing on the treadmill, cycling

Follow-Up

After three weeks, B.L. is able to participate in endurance exercise at a rating of per-ceived exertion of 10/20 during 10 minutes of continuous brisk walking on the treadmill (see Chapter 4). She is able to complete a full yoga class without experiencing fatigue and taking a break. B.L. uses a fitness app on her phone to keep track of her exer-cise minutes and enjoys sharing her program with other friends logging their minutes.

The authors would like to acknowledge Kara Tischer, PT, DPT, for her contribu-tions to the case study.

References

American College of Sports Medicine. (2014). *ACSM's guidelines for exercising testing and prescrip-tion* (9th ed.). Philadelphia, PA: Wolters Kluwer Health/Lippincott Williams & Wilkins.

Blaney, J.M., Lowe-Strong, A., Rankin-Watt, J., Campbell, A., & Gracey, J.H. (2013). Cancer survivors' exercise barriers, facilitators and preferences in the context of fatigue, quality of life and physical activity participation: A questionnaire–survey. *Psycho-Oncology, 22,* 186–194. doi:10.1002/pon.2072

Brant, J.M., & Wickham, R. (Eds.). (2013). *Statement on the scope and standards of oncology nursing practice: Generalist and advanced practice.* Pittsburgh, PA: Oncology Nursing Society.

Cadmus-Bertram, L.A., Marcus, B.H., Patterson, R.E., Parker, B.A., & Morey, B.L. (2015). Randomized trial of a Fitbit-based physical activity intervention for women. *American Journal of Preventive Medicine, 49,* 414–418. doi:10.1016/j.amepre.2015.01.020

National Comprehensive Cancer Network. (2016). *NCCN Clinical Practice Guidelines in Oncology (NCCN Guidelines®): Cancer-related fatigue* [v.1.2016]. Retrieved from https://www.nccn.org/professionals/physician_gls/pdf/fatigue.pdf

Schmitz, K.H., Courneya, K.S., Matthews, C., Demark-Wahnefried, W., Galvão, D.A., Pinto, B.M., ... Schwartz, A.L. (2010). American College of Sports Medicine roundtable on exercise guidelines for cancer survivors. *Medicine and Science in Sports and Exercise, 42,* 1409–1426. doi:10.1249/MSS.0b013e3181e0c112

Stevinson, C., Lawlor, D.A., & Fox, K.R. (2004). Exercise interventions for cancer patients: Systematic review of controlled trials. *Cancer Causes and Control, 15,* 1035–1056. doi:10.1007/s10552-004-1325-4

Van Gerpen, R.E., & Becker, B.J. (2013). Development of an evidence-based exercise and education cancer recovery program. *Clinical Journal of Oncology Nursing, 17,* 539–543. doi:10.1188/13.CJON.539-543

CHAPTER 8

Physical Activity for Cancer-Related Fatigue

Jean Godfroy, RN, BSN, CBCN®, OCN®, and Julie Griffie, RN, MSN, AOCN®

Introduction

Cancer-related fatigue (CRF) is recognized as one of the most frequently experienced side effects of cancer and its treatment (Bower, 2014). Best defined as a distressing, persistent subjective sense of physical, emotional, or cognitive tiredness or exhaustion related to cancer

> *"My whole being is tired. I am overwhelmed by the simple desire to not do things. Changing the toilet paper roll or even flushing the toilet seems like a huge effort. Simple things I have always taken for granted are now major efforts. It's just total physical and emotional tiredness."*
>
> —A patient

or cancer treatment, CRF is not proportional to recent activity and interferes with usual functioning (Bower et al., 2014; Howell et al., 2013; National Comprehensive Cancer Network® [NCCN®], 2016). CRF may increase and decrease in the course of the day and follow patterns related to the administration of treatments. CRF may be difficult to distinguish from depression.

Reports of fatigue span the trajectory of diagnosis, treatment, and end-of-life care. Cancer survivors describe it as "overwhelming," "relentless," and "unrelieved by rest." CRF often is feared as a sign that treatment is not going well. Pain, sleep disturbances, and cognitive functioning issues may influence fatigue.

Although physical activity and exercise can help ameliorate the effects of CRF, cancer survivors may not want to stay active when they are tired. Oncology nurses may find that cancer survivors in the midst of their fatigue experience find it hard to understand that physical activity and exercise improve their quality of life and relieve fatigue, simply because it may seem counterintuitive. However, exercise is a useful strategy for managing fatigue, as well as improving health-related quality of life, including physical, role, and social functions (Mishra, Scherer, Snyder, Geigle, & Gotay, 2015). Therefore, oncology nurses can take a proactive stance by educating cancer survivors before, during, and after treatment on safe and effective ways to remain physically active.

This chapter describes the etiology of CRF, as well as the positive effects that physical activity and exercise have on fatigue. Screening and assessment measures for CRF applicable to oncology nursing practice are presented. The FITT principle (see Chapter 4) is applied to assist oncology nurses in the creation and evaluation of physical activities and exercises that can help with fatigue. Oncology nurses can incorporate this chapter's content to create individualized plans of care to promote physical activities that reduce or ameliorate CRF in cancer survivors. These plans address the activity goals recommended by NCCN (2016) and the American College of Sports Medicine (ACSM) (see Figure 8-1) (Schmitz et al., 2010). This chapter's content is supported in the Oncology Nursing Society's (ONS's) *Statement on the Scope and Standards of Oncology Nursing Practice: Generalist and Advanced Practice* (Brant & Wickham, 2013) (see Figure 8-2).

- Fatigue should be screened, assessed, and managed according to clinical practice guidelines.
- Encourage patients to engage in a moderate level of physical activity during and after cancer treatment. The exercise program should be individualized based on the patient's age, gender, type of cancer, and physical fitness level.
- Consider cancer-specific exercise programs if available. The program should begin at a low level of intensity and duration, progress slowly, and be modified as the patient's condition changes.
- Evidence suggests that exercise is beneficial to individuals with incurable cancer and short life expectancy, although it is important to consider patients' physical constraints.
- Exercise is effective in reducing the burden of several specific cancers, including demonstrated benefits related to physical function, quality of life, and cancer-related fatigue.
- Patients should avoid inactivity.
- Patients should return to normal daily activity as soon as possible following surgery.
- Patients may continue normal daily activities and exercise as much as possible during and after nonsurgical treatments.

Figure 8-1. Clinical Guidelines for Cancer-Related Fatigue

Note. Based on information from National Comprehensive Cancer Network, 2016.

Cancer-Related Fatigue

Fatigue must be treated across the broad spectrum of what it is: a multidimensional phenomenon with mechanisms that result in a decreased capacity for mental as well as physical work (Jacobsen, 2004). No clear agreement exists

Standard I. Assessment
- Collect data in the following high-incidence problem areas. These areas may include but are not limited to the following:
  - Comfort: Location, intensity, quality, temporal, and exacerbating and relieving characteristics of discomfort/pain and other deleterious symptoms (e.g., fatigue, nausea, dyspnea, rash, pruritus); nonverbal rating scales for patients who are unable to communicate the presence of symptoms
  - Mobility
    * Past and present level of mobility and overall function
    * Risk for decreased mobility
    * Impact of fatigue on mobility
    * Complications related to decreased mobility
  - Survivorship
    * Patient/family understanding of the potential late effects of cancer treatment (e.g., secondary malignancies, organ toxicities, altered fertility, osteoporosis) prior to initiation of therapy
    * Patient/family understanding of the potential persistent or long-term effects associated with cancer treatment (e.g., fatigue, taste changes, cognitive changes, osteoporosis)

Standard II. Diagnosis
- Use evidence-based research to formulate the plan of care.

Standard III. Outcome Identification
- Develop expected outcomes for each of the high-incidence problem areas at a level consistent with the patient's physical, psychological, social, and spiritual capacities, cultural background, and value system. The expected outcomes include but are not limited to the following:
  - Comfort: Describe appropriate interventions for potential or predictable problems, such as pain, fatigue, dyspnea, sleep pattern disturbances, nausea, vomiting, and pruritus.
  - Mobility: The patient and/or family
    * Incorporate safety and fall prevention strategies in the mobility plan.
    * Explain the impact of fatigue on immobility.
    * Explain the relationship between fatigue and exercise balance.
    * Describe an appropriate management plan to integrate alteration in mobility into lifestyle.
    * Describe optimal levels of activities of daily living at a level consistent with disease state and treatment.
    * Identify health services and community resources available for managing changes in mobility.
    * Use assistive devices to aid or improve mobility.
    * Demonstrate measures to prevent the complications of decreased mobility (e.g., pressure ulcers, pneumonia).

Figure 8-2. Standards Applicable to Physical Activity for Reducing Cancer-Related Fatigue

(Continued on next page)

Standard IV. Planning
• Develop the plan of care in collaboration with the patient, family, interdisciplinary cancer care team, and other healthcare professionals when possible.

Standard V. Implementation
• Use evidence-based research to guide implementation of interventions.

Standard VI. Evaluation
• Communicate the patient's response with the interdisciplinary cancer care team and other agencies involved in the healthcare continuum.

Figure 8-2. Standards Applicable to Physical Activity for Reducing Cancer-Related Fatigue (Continued)

Note. From *Statement on the Scope and Standards of Oncology Nursing Practice: Generalist and Advanced Practice,* by J.M. Brant and R. Wickham (Eds.), 2013, Pittsburgh, PA: Oncology Nursing Society. Copyright 2013 by Oncology Nursing Society. Adapted with permission.

on the etiology and pathogenesis of fatigue, and it is not explained by physiologic mechanisms alone. Commonly hypothesized models to explain CRF have been presented (Bower, 2014; Meriggi, 2014; O'Neil-Page, Anderson, & Dean, 2015). Fatigue is influenced by a multitude of factors (see Figure 8-3).
• Accumulation hypothesis: Waste products build up faster than the body can eliminate them, resulting in fatigue.
• Concept of depletion: Elements essential to body function become unavailable.
• Concept of deregulation of the proinflammatory cytokines network: In humans, proinflammatory cytokines are thought to be released in response to infection, tumor, tissue damage, or the depletion of immune cells.
• Serotonin increase: Increased levels occur in the presence of tumor growth and treatment.

Benefits of Physical Activity and Exercise on Cancer-Related Fatigue

Physical activity and exercise have been recognized as interventions that favorably impact CRF (Bower et al., 2014; Howell et al., 2013; Jose & Diwan, 2014; Mishra, Scherer, Snyder, Geigle, & Gotay, 2014; Mitchell et al., 2014; Schmitz et al., 2010). ONS's Putting Evidence Into Practice (PEP) resource on CRF management confirms physical activity and exercise as the only recommended practice intervention for the management of CRF (Irwin, Poirier, & Mitchell, 2014; Mitchell et al., 2014). Furthermore, the 2010 ACSM roundtable supports the ONS PEP resource, recommending that cancer survivors avoid inactivity and move as their ability and condition allow (Schmitz et al., 2010). In a meta-analysis conducted by Puetz and Herring (2012), exercise reduced levels of CRF in patients during and after treatment. Exercise was described to

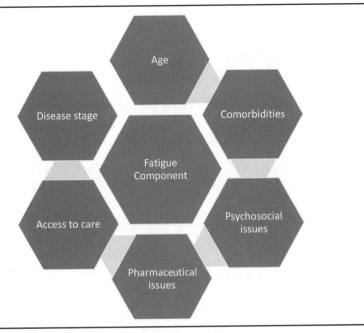

Figure 8-3. Multifactorial Components of Fatigue

Note. Based on information from Jacobsen, 2004.

have a palliative effect on CRF during treatment and a rehabilitative effect following treatment. NCCN (2016) recommends physical activity, based on ability, throughout the cancer trajectory (i.e., during and after treatment).

Cardiovascular Exercise

In their meta-analysis of 56 studies involving 4,068 cancer survivors, Cramp and Byron-Daniel (2012) found that aerobic/cardiovascular exercise reduces fatigue during and after cancer treatment, particularly for breast and prostate cancer survivors. The most frequent cardiovascular exercises were walking and cycling.

Walking is an exercise that is easily undertaken by most cancer survivors because the intensity (pace, incline) and time are discretionary. Helping to procure a safe walking environment is an important step in creating a walking program. Griffie and Godfroy (2014) reported the challenges surrounding the implementation of a walking track in an oncology clinic setting. Successful implementation required having the multidisciplinary team answer questions such as the following:

• What is the program's standard for self-report and assessment of CRF?
• Can nurses suggest that patients exercise without a written order?

• When should a referral to physical therapy be made?
• What multimodality interventions (e.g., yoga, structural dimensional rehabilitation such as psychoeducation, nutrition counseling, massage, relaxation) are available and can be implemented by the nurse?
• Can walking be suggested for every patient?
• What community resource referrals can be initiated by the nurse?

The multidisciplinary team defined clinical criteria for when nurses could recommend exercise regimens (per nursing judgment). The criteria for nurse recommendation included patients who were receiving adjuvant therapy, had normal hemoglobin and hematocrit levels, were afebrile, had no known metastatic disease or cognitive impairments, and had performance status scores within normal limits. The walking track implementation helped demonstrate to patients that walking was an easy and valued way to incorporate physical activity into daily routines as well as during their required time in the clinic setting.

Strength/Endurance Exercise

Cramp and Byron-Daniel's (2012) meta-analysis found that strength/endurance exercise was not associated with improved fatigue in cancer survivors. However, strength/endurance activities should be included as part of survivors' daily physical activities to promote muscle strength, bone strength, bal-

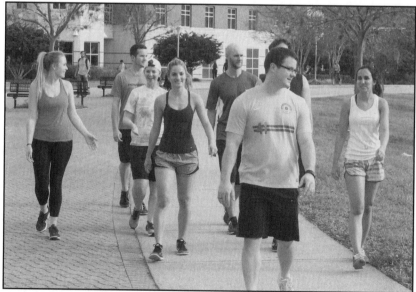

Walking is a form of exercise that is self-paced and can be completed in a variety of settings.

ance, and coordination. Examples of daily strength/endurance activities include lifting items such as cans of food, laundry, and pots and pans and walking on an incline, such as up a flight of stairs.

Flexibility Exercise

Cramp and Byron-Daniel's (2012) meta-analysis found that flexibility exercise was not associated with improved fatigue in cancer survivors. However, flexibility activities should be included as part of survivors' daily physical activities to promote joint mobility and muscle lengthening. Examples of daily flexibility include reaching for items such as cans of food, dishes, and clothing; turning to fasten a seat belt; and stretching in bed upon awakening.

Oncology Nursing Assessment

A standard documentation tool for fatigue assessment should be used by oncology nurses in the outpatient clinic, infusion area, inpatient area, and therapy area. Scores, assessment data, and current outcomes of interventions should be available in flow sheet format for easy comparison across treatment sites. Documentation of the fatigue assessment must be viewable by the oncology team and other healthcare professionals involved in the survivor's treatment across the healthcare continuum. Validated fatigue assessment scales have been reviewed and found to be useful in research and everyday clinical use (Borneman, 2013; Minton & Stone, 2009; Seyidova-Khoshknabi, Davis, & Walsh, 2011). Fatigue assessment scales must be practical for application in a busy oncology practice, therapy clinic, and inpatient area.

Organizational effort must be made to ensure that documentation tools reflect national standards. Figure 8-4 provides an example of a documentation tool for fatigue self-report and assessment in an electronic medical record. In addition to the cancer survivor's self-report of fatigue, content for documentation from the National Cancer Institute Cancer Therapy Evaluation Program (2010) Common Terminology Criteria for Adverse Events (CTCAE) is contained in the choices for documentation. CTCAE criteria were developed for the purpose of standardizing the classification of adverse effects of drugs used in cancer therapy. The criteria are commonly required in the assessments of patients participating in clinical research trials. Oncology nurses and clinical research coordinators must use the same terminology so that there is consistency in fatigue (and other toxicity or side effect) assessments. Fatigue descriptors can be found online under General Disorders in the CTCAE compilation. The cancer survivor's subjective report of fatigue should be captured in a standard scale that can be used and retrieved for comparison across the organization's settings (see Figure 8-4).

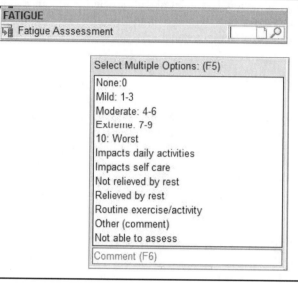

Figure 8-4. Documentation Tool for Fatigue Self-Report and Assessment in an Electronic Medical Record

Note. Copyright 2015 by Epic Systems Corporation. Used with permission.

Self-Report and Fatigue Assessment Measures

1. Obtain a baseline assessment for fatigue. Screening for fatigue begins at the time of cancer diagnosis. At minimum, a baseline assessment for fatigue must include the following:
   • Report of fatigue
   • Physical assessment
   • Information on current routine physical activity
   • Performance status
2. After the baseline assessment, assess for fatigue at predetermined intervals, as clinically indicated, and on an annual basis (Bower et al., 2014).
3. After treatment commencement, assess for fatigue at each clinic visit. Determine the effects of drug or radiation toxicities on self-reported fatigue.
4. After treatment completion, assess for fatigue when the survivorship care plan is reviewed (Rowland & Bellizzi, 2014).
5. Assess for fatigue using self-report and established screening measures.
   • The NCCN (2015a) Distress Thermometer (see Figure 8-5) is a self-assessment tool that captures the distress that cancer survivors may be experiencing regarding ongoing issues (e.g., family, financial, emotional, physical issues; spiritual concerns).

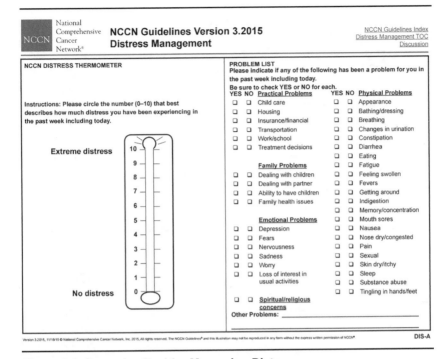

Figure 8-5. Screening Tool for Measuring Distress

Note. Reproduced with permission from *NCCN Clinical Practice Guidelines in Oncology (NCCN Guidelines®) for Distress Management V.1.2015.* © 2015 by the National Comprehensive Cancer Network, Inc. All rights reserved. The NCCN Guidelines® and illustrations herein may not be reproduced in any form for any purpose without the express written permission of the NCCN. To view the most recent and complete version of the NCCN Guidelines, go online to NCCN.org. NATIONAL COMPREHENSIVE CANCER NETWORK®, NCCN®, NCCN GUIDELINES®, and all other NCCN Content are trademarks owned by the National Comprehensive Cancer Network, Inc.

- A visual analog scale (VAS) contains images representing degrees of fatigue placed over a numeric range of scores (see Figure 8-6). The pictures assist survivors in translating the image to a score. Individuals use the tool to score their fatigue using a numeric scale ranging from 0 (no fatigue) to 10 (worst fatigue), as it relates to the pictures. Figure 8-7 shows a VAS used for individuals who speak English, Spanish, Arabic, Mandarin, and Vietnamese (Vispacom, Inc., 2012). Figures 8-6 and 8-7 use the same numeric scale, and both are designed to facilitate patient–provider communication.
- The Brief Fatigue Inventory (BFI) assesses severe fatigue (see Figure 8-8). The BFI is simple and easy to use and takes approximately five minutes to complete. The tool provides information on six fatigue interface items: general activity, mood, walking ability, normal work, relations with others, and

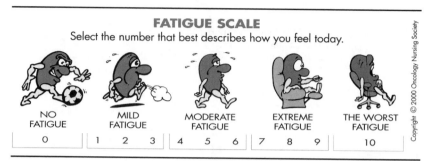

Figure 8-6. Visual Analog Scale to Rate Fatigue

Note. Copyright 2000 by Oncology Nursing Society. Used with permission.

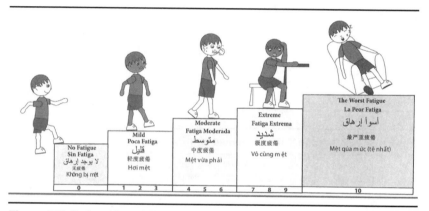

Figure 8-7. Fatigue Level Chart

Note. Copyright 2012 by E. Garcia, Vispacom LLC. Used with permission.

enjoyment of life. The BFI was noted as a nonburdensome tool in patients with advanced stages of cancer (Seyidova-Khoshknabi et al., 2011).

6. Interpret self-report fatigue scores:
   • Mild fatigue = 1–3
   • Moderate fatigue = 4–6
   • Severe fatigue = 7–10
7. Evaluate the self-reported fatigue score with the following considerations:
   • Rating fatigue from 0 to 10 may be overwhelming for cancer survivors.
   • Survivors may have difficulty self-scoring and find it hard to conceptualize a number without an image of what that means to their personal situation.
   • Survivors may minimize their self-report score as well as the importance of it to their provider.

Brief Fatigue Inventory

STUDY ID# _____   HOSPITAL # _____

Date: _____ / _____ / _____   Time: _____

Name _____ _____ _____
        Last   First   Middle Initial

Throughout our lives, most of us have times when we feel very tired or fatigued. Have you felt unusually tired or fatigued in the last week? Yes ▮   No ▮

1. Please rate your fatigue (weariness, tiredness) by circling the one number that best describes your fatigue right NOW.

0	1	2	3	4	5	6	7	8	9	10
No Fatigue										As bad as you can imagine

2. Please rate your fatigue (weariness, tiredness) by circling the one number that best describes your USUAL level of fatigue during past 24 hours.

0	1	2	3	4	5	6	7	8	9	10
No Fatigue										As bad as you can imagine

3. Please rate your fatigue (weariness, tiredness) by circling the one number that best describes your WORST level of fatigue during past 24 hours.

0	1	2	3	4	5	6	7	8	9	10
No Fatigue										As bad as you can imagine

4. Circle the one number that describes how, during the past 24 hours, fatigue has interfered with your:

A. General activity

0	1	2	3	4	5	6	7	8	9	10
Does not interfere										Completely Interferes

B. Mood

0	1	2	3	4	5	6	7	8	9	10
Does not interfere										Completely Interferes

C. Walking ability

0	1	2	3	4	5	6	7	8	9	10
Does not interfere										Completely Interferes

D. Normal work (includes both work outside the home and daily chores)

0	1	2	3	4	5	6	7	8	9	10
Does not interfere										Completely Interferes

E. Relations with other people

0	1	2	3	4	5	6	7	8	9	10
Does not interfere										Completely Interferes

F. Enjoyment of life

0	1	2	3	4	5	6	7	8	9	10
Does not interfere										Completely Interferes

Figure 8-8. Brief Fatigue Inventory

8. Obtain a history and physical examination, including laboratory evaluation, on cancer survivors who self-report moderate to severe fatigue (score of 4–10) prior to discussing physical activities and exercises.

9. Obtain your oncology center's current fatigue assessment scales. Review your center's fatigue assessment scales and compare them with the scales listed in this chapter.

10. Assess for fatigue-specific parameters such as the following:
    - Fatigue onset
    - Fatigue duration
    - Exacerbating and palliating factors
    - Treatments tried to help with fatigue
    - Barriers to interventions

11. Assess for treatment-related fatigue parameters such as the following (American Cancer Society, 2014):
    - Tiredness that does not get better
    - Tiredness that keeps coming back or gets worst
    - Tiredness not related to activity
    - Tiredness that does not get better with rest or sleep
    - Increased need for sleep
    - Confusion
    - Inability to concentrate or focus
    - Survivor in bed for more than 24 hours
    - Tiredness that disrupts work, social life, or daily routines
    - Lack of desire to do normal things
    - Feelings of sadness, depression, or irritability

Self-Report and Physical Activity/Exercise Assessment

1. Assess survivors' current physical activity and exercise patterns using measures such as those described in Chapter 4. Use the physical activity and exercise measures endorsed by your oncology center to measure activity. Assessing cancer survivors' current physical activity and exercise programs will make it easier to understand the level of physical activity in which they are currently engaged.

2. Evaluate the relationship between survivors' physical activity and self-reported fatigue. Use the FITT principle (see Chapter 4) to assess the frequency, intensity, time, and type of activities. Are the types of activities performed at too high of an intensity (> 6 metabolic equivalent of tasks [METs]) or too frequently? Is there a balance of strength and flexibility activities? Are aerobic/cardiovascular activities included in the daily activities?

3. Use screenings (see Chapter 6) as needed to determine physical readiness for exercise.

4. Determine if a consultation to a physical or occupational therapist is indicated if debilitation is observed (see Chapter 12).

Oncology Nursing Recommendations for Physical Activity and Exercise to Manage Fatigue

1. Use any of the interviewing techniques discussed in Chapter 5 to determine survivors' readiness to incorporate physical activity and exercise into their lifestyle.
2. Teach survivors about fatigue through written information. Be sure to include the following information:
   - Fatigue is a common side effect of treatment. Because fatigue is often perceived to be an indication of treatment failure, this concern should be addressed clearly at the beginning of treatment and reinforced as indicated.
   - Report the inability to do normal activities and/or if still very tired after resting or sleeping. Self-report should be done as fatigue occurs and not delayed until the next appointment.
   - Accomplish the most important tasks first. Don't pack too many activities into the day.
   - Drink eight glasses of water per day. Five to six small meals may be easier to tolerate than three large meals.
   - Rest when needed.
   - If helpful, nap for one hour or less during the day.
   - Establish a bedtime routine (e.g., bathing, reading, listening to music) to help relax at night (see Chapter 11).
3. Teach survivors about the potential benefits of physical activity and exercise on fatigue. Use the evidence presented in this chapter to create a patient education fact sheet. Use the education materials provided by your oncology center. Assure them that an individualized physical activity and exercise plan have been shown to be safe for helping to reduce fatigue during and after cancer treatment.
4. Use interventions to reduce CRF, including those recommended by ONS PEP resources (Irwin et al., 2014) (see Chapter 15).
5. Collaborate with survivors to select physical activities and exercises they enjoy and are able to perform regularly and safely. Use checklists offered by your oncology center or the lists provided in Chapters 1 and 4.
6. Use the FITT principle to collaborate with survivors and create a physical activity and exercise plan. For CRF, physical activity and exercise are based on survivors' baseline activity level. Unless contraindicated, encourage survivors to maintain their current activity level. The following is an example of a physical activity program for survivors experiencing fatigue (Mitchell et al., 2014):
   - Frequency: Twice a day
   - Intensity: Two laps around track, pacing based on level of fatigue
   - Time: 5–10 minutes (increase by one minute each day)
   - Type: Walking

7. Consider chemotherapy treatment schedules, blood counts, surgery-related restrictions, and other health-related factors when creating a physical activity plan. For fatigue, the plan should be scaled based on daily self-reported fatigue.

8. Calculate the target heart rate zone by using the Karvonen formula. Teach survivors how to measure their heart rate and measure their rating of perceived exertion (RPE) (see Chapter 7).

9. Encourage cancer survivors who are not participating in physical activity to adopt the program created with their oncology nurse. Encourage family participation in the plan. Offer energy conservation tips to help cancer survivors adhere to and stay engaged in activity. Encourage strategies such as the following:
   • Consolidate trips up and down stairs.
   • Wash dishes once a day only or use paper plates.
   • Sit when doing tasks that involve using upper extremities.

10. Provide survivors with a discharge packet for physical activity to help reduce fatigue that includes the following information:
    • RPE during endurance exercise (Borg rating scale)
    • Calculated target heart rate during each endurance exercise (Karvonen formula)
    • FITT principle–based physical activity and exercise plan for fatigue
    • Self-report fatigue scale (visual or numeric) used by your oncology center

11. Set short-term (daily or weekly) and long-term (monthly) goals with survivors and their families for physical activity and exercise to gradually reach 150 minutes of aerobic activity per week (Jankowski & Matthews, 2011).

12. Encourage survivors to report moderate to severe symptoms after starting physical activity and exercise in order to discuss ways to reduce these symptoms.

13. Select a method for tracking physical activity and fatigue levels. Personal tracking devices are available that monitor physical activity and heart rate and interface with a computer or mobile app to provide feedback on distance and heart rate while giving survivors control and quick feedback on their performance. Many aspects of activity can be monitored and graphed for individuals wanting details. Such personal tracking devices must be safe, fit the individual's lifestyle, and be practical. Ask survivors to bring the tracking device with them on their next visit.

14. Recommend support systems, such as a walking partner or group, and resources, including indoor walking facilities, to initiate and maintain an active physical activity and exercise plan.

15. Provide resources related to CRF:
    • The National Cancer Institute provides fatigue education for patients undergoing chemotherapy and for patients receiving radiation therapy.
    • ONS provides patient education on evidence-based fatigue interventions for CRF.
    • NCCN provides guidelines for survivorship (NCCN, 2015b).

Oncology Nursing Evaluation of Health Outcomes

1. Evaluate cancer survivors' adherence to their recommended physical activity/exercise plan by discussing their self-report outcomes (see Chapter 7).
2. Evaluate these outcomes to the plan adherence and self-reported fatigue. Note any effects on fatigue levels and ratings.
3. Discuss survivors' experiences with the physical activity and exercise plan as well as their fatigue patterns. Use the interviewing techniques in Chapter 5.
4. Revise the physical activity and exercise plans as needed. Adjust the frequency, intensity, time, and type of activities to meet survivors' needs.
5. Follow up with referrals for physical or occupational therapy and for exercise testing as required by your oncology center.

Application to Oncology Nursing Practice

1. Fatigue is rarely an isolated symptom. The information provided by cancer survivors allows oncology nurses to intervene in situations that may easily be remedied or resolved, resulting in improved outcomes. Standards for fatigue evaluation have been defined by the American Society of Clinical Oncology and NCCN and can be found throughout the literature (Bower et al., 2014; Howell et al., 2013; NCCN, 2016).
2. Analyzing cancer survivors' self-reports of fatigue, along with their psychosocial and physical readiness for physical activity and exercise, allows oncology nurses to determine the best approach for creating a doable activity plan. The activity plan is tailored to fit the fatigue patterns experienced by cancer survivors; for example, when fatigue is high, activities with high METs (see Chapter 2) and intensity should be limited (see Chapter 4).
3. Oncology nurses and cancer survivors can use the FITT principle to create an achievable physical activity plan. Evaluating the effects of the recommended physical activity plan on CRF at subsequent visits allows oncology nurses to measure the effect of physical activity on cancer survivors' self-reported fatigue.

Summary

Fatigue is rarely an isolated symptom. The oncology nurse's ability to understand the causes of survivor distress and provide interventions and support for resolution should result in improved patient outcomes. Oncology nurses are charged with assessing, educating, and planning interventions that assist individuals in managing CRF and recognizing when additional healthcare team members should be consulted. The unique and complex dynamic of each person's fatigue experience should be explored routinely.

Exercise and physical activity are the most successful fatigue management interventions to date. However, exercise does not result in quick changes. Fatigue management strategies must be adjusted throughout a survivor's life. Until further knowledge of the etiology of CRF is known, oncology nurses' clinical judgement, survivors' assessment factors and preferences, and best evidence should determine the plan of care specific to each cancer survivor.

Case Study

M.N. is a 72-year-old woman who is a five-year survivor of breast cancer. M.N. previously followed exercise and nutrition recommendations for her age; yoga and walking were big parts of M.N.'s life prior to diagnosis and treatment.

M.N. attends church and has a group of friends with whom she attends church activities. She also serves as the primary caregiver for her chronically ill husband. M.N. reports a fatigue score of 7/10 that limits her ability to cook meals and carry out daily activities. Prior to treatment, her self-rated fatigue score was 0/10, and her distress scale score was 4/10. She states that fatigue is worse approximately 17 hours after pegfilgrastim injections.

M.N. requires naps every day. Her treatment plan includes neoadjuvant chemotherapy with the goal of lumpectomy, followed by radiation therapy and trastuzumab for a year. Neoadjuvant chemotherapy consists of TCH (docetaxel, carboplatin, and trastuzumab).

Loratadine is ordered in place of pegfilgrastim, along with a dose reduction of pegfilgrastim. M.N. responds well, and her fatigue score is reduced to 5/10 following her fourth treatment cycle. M.N. is also referred to a nutritionist (see Figure 8-9).

Relevant Laboratory Values
All within normal limits.

Energy Conservation Techniques
- Seek assistance from church friends in preparing meals.
- Utilize disposable plates and utensils to reduce time and effort of loading and unloading dishwasher or washing dishes by hand.
- Seek help from family members or church friends to assist with husband's care when necessary.
- When overwhelmed with treatment and side effects, remember the three D's: delay, delete, and delegate.

Height/weight	• Height: 5'6" • Weight: 142 lbs • BMI: 23 • Healthy weight
Vitals	• Blood pressure: 118/79 mm Hg • Resting heart rate: 80 bpm • Temperature: 98.6°F (37°C)
Cardiopulmonary	• Normal breath sounds bilaterally • Normal cardiovascular examination

Figure 8-9. Additional Patient Information

BMI—body mass index; bpm—beats per minute

Sample Initial Exercise Prescription				
Exercise Type	**Frequency**	**Intensity**	**Time**	**Type**
Strength training	2 days per week to tolerance in home	Body weight	10–15 minutes	Strength yoga
Cardiovascular	3 days per week	Light to start (up to 50% maximum heart rate or rating of perceived exertion [RPE] of 2–3/10) Individual should be able to easily talk during exercise without feeling out of breath (see Table 4-3 in Chapter 4).	10-minute intervals, working up to 30 minutes of sustained exercise	Walking
Flexibility	Warm-up and cooldown with aerobic exercise	Low load to the point of resistance	5–10 minutes	Stretching
	2 days per week to tolerance in home	Position at the point of resistance; no more than mild discomfort	10–15 minutes	Yoga
Sample Moderate Exercise Progression				
Strength training and balance	2–3 days per week	Body weight	55 minutes	Yoga
Cardiovascular	5–7 days per week	Moderate physical exertion or 50%–70% maximum heart rate or RPE of 4/10	45–60 minutes	Brisk walking

(Continued on next page)

Sample Initial Exercise Prescription *(Continued)*				
Exercise Type	Frequency	Intensity	Time	Type
Flexibility	Warm-up and cooldown	Low load to the point of resistance	5–10 minutes	Stretching
	2 days per week to tolerance in home	Position at the point of resistance; no more than mild discomfort	20–30 minutes	Flexibility yoga

Follow-Up

Six months following completion of radiation treatment, M.N. is able to increase her exercise tolerance (duration and intensity) slowly throughout treatment. She also is able to resume age-recommended activity levels. M.N. attributes her success to the encouragement of her nurses and doctors to continue being active. Her self-reported fatigue score was 2/10 following treatment and continues to improve.

Twelve months following completion of radiation treatment, M.N. is on an aromatase inhibitor that causes her joint pain. She learns to take it in the morning and stays busy and active so that the pain is not so noticeable and more tolerable.

References

American Cancer Society. (2014). Fatigue in people with cancer. Retrieved from http://www.cancer.org/acs/groups/cid/documents/webcontent/002842-pdf.pdf

Borneman, T. (2013). Assessment and management of cancer-related fatigue. *Journal of Hospice and Palliative Nursing, 15*, 77–86. doi:10.1097/NJH.0b013e318286dc19

Bower, J.E. (2014). Cancer-related fatigue—Mechanisms, risk factors, and treatments. *Nature Reviews Clinical Oncology, 11*, 597–609. doi:10.1038/nrclinonc.2014.127

Bower, J.E., Bak, K., Berger, A., Breitbart, W., Escalante, C.P., Ganz, P.A., ... Jacobsen, P.B. (2014). Screening, assessment, and management of fatigue in adult survivors of cancer: An American Society of Clinical Oncology clinical practice guideline adaptation. *Journal of Clinical Oncology, 32*, 1840–1850. doi:10.1200/JCO.2013.53.4495

Brant, J.M., & Wickham, R. (Eds.). (2013). *Statement on the scope and standards of oncology nursing practice: Generalist and advanced practice.* Pittsburgh, PA: Oncology Nursing Society.

Cramp, F., & Byron-Daniel, J. (2012). Exercise for the management of cancer-related fatigue in adults. *Cochrane Database of Systematic Reviews, 2012*(11). doi:10.1002/14651858.CD006145.pub3

Griffie, J., & Godfroy, J. (2014). Improving cancer-related fatigue outcomes: Walking patients through treatment and beyond. *Clinical Journal of Oncology Nursing, 18*(Suppl. 5), 21–24. doi:10.1188/14.CJON.S2.21-24

Howell, D., Keller-Olaman, S., Oliver, T.K., Hack, T.F., Broadfield, L., Biggs, K., ... Olson, K. (2013). A pan-Canadian practice guideline and algorithm: Screening, assessment, and supportive care of adults with cancer-related fatigue. *Current Oncology, 20*, E233–E246. doi:10.3747/co.20.1302

Irwin, M., Poirier, P., & Mitchell, S.A. (2014). Fatigue. In M. Irwin & L.A. Johnson (Eds.), *Putting evidence into practice: A pocket guide to cancer symptom management* (pp. 111–122). Pittsburgh, PA: Oncology Nursing Society.

Jacobsen, P.B. (2004). Assessment of fatigue in cancer patients. *Journal of the National Cancer Institute Monographs, 2004*(32), 93–97. doi:10.1093/jncimonographs/lgh010

Jankowski, C.M., & Matthews, E.E. (2011). Exercise guidelines for adults with cancer: A vital role in survivorship. *Clinical Journal of Oncology Nursing, 15,* 683–686. doi:10.1188/11.CJON.683-686

Jose, S., & Diwan, S.K. (2014). Effect of standardized exercise program on reported fatigue in patients of cancer receiving chemotherapy. *Clinical Cancer Investigation Journal, 3,* 373–376. doi:10.4103/2278-0513.138053

Meriggi, R. (2014). Cancer-related fatigue: Still an enigma to be solved quickly. *Reviews on Recent Clinical Trials, 9,* 267–270. doi:10.2174/1574887109666141127111008

Minton, O., & Stone, P. (2009). A systematic review of the scales used for the measurement of cancer-related fatigue (CRF). *Annals of Oncology, 20,* 17–25. doi:10.1093/annonc/mdn537

Mishra, S.I., Scherer, R.W., Snyder, C., Geigle, P., & Gotay, C. (2014). Are exercise programs effective for improving health-related quality of life among cancer survivors? A systematic review and meta-analysis [Online exclusive]. *Oncology Nursing Forum, 41,* E326–E342. doi:10.1188/14.ONF.E326-E342

Mishra, S.I., Scherer, R.W., Snyder, C., Geigle, P., & Gotay, C. (2015). The effectiveness of exercise interventions for improving health-related quality of life from diagnosis through active cancer treatment [Online exclusive]. *Oncology Nursing Forum, 42,* E33–E53. doi:10.1188/15.ONF.E33-E53

Mitchell, S.A., Hoffman, A.J., Clark, J.C., DeGennaro, R.M., Poirier, P., Robinson, C.B., & Weisbrod, B.L. (2014). Putting evidence into practice: An update of evidence-based interventions for cancer-related fatigue during and following treatment. *Clinical Journal of Oncology Nursing, 18*(Suppl. 6), 38–58. doi:10.1188/14.CJON.S3.38-58

National Cancer Institute Cancer Therapy Evaluation Program. (2010). *Common terminology criteria for adverse events* [v.4.03]. Retrieved from http://evs.nci.nih.gov/ftp1/CTCAE/CTCAE_4.03_2010-06-14_QuickReference_8.5x11.pdf

National Comprehensive Cancer Network. (2015a). *NCCN Clinical Practice Guidelines in Oncology (NCCN Guidelines®): Distress management* [v.1.2015]. Retrieved from http://www.nccn.org/professionals/physician_gls/pdf/distress.pdf

National Comprehensive Cancer Network. (2015b). *NCCN Clinical Practice Guidelines in Oncology (NCCN Guidelines®): Survivorship* [v.2.2015]. Retrieved from http://www.nccn.org/professionals/physician_gls/pdf/survivorship

National Comprehensive Cancer Network. (2016). *NCCN Clinical Practice Guidelines in Oncology: (NCCN Guidelines®) Cancer-related fatigue* [v.1.2016]. Retrieved from http://www.nccn.org/professionals/physician_gls/pdf/fatigue.pdf

O'Neil-Page, E., Anderson, P.R., & Dean, G.E. (2015). Fatigue. In B.R. Ferrell, N. Coyle, & J. Paice (Eds.), *Oxford textbook of palliative nursing* (4th ed., pp. 154–166). New York, NY: Oxford University Press.

Puetz, T.W., & Herring, M.P. (2012). Differential effects of exercise on cancer-related fatigue during and following treatment: A meta-analysis. *American Journal of Preventive Medicine, 43*(2), E1–E24. doi:10.1016/j.amepre.2012.04.027

Rowland, J.H., & Bellizzi, K.M. (2014). Cancer survivorship issues: Life after treatment and implications for an aging population. *Journal of Clinical Oncology, 32,* 2662–2668. doi:10.1200/JCO.2014.55.8361

Schmitz, K.H., Courneya, K.S., Matthews, C., Demark-Wahnefried, W., Galvão, D.A., Pinto, B.M., ... Schwartz, A.L. (2010). American College of Sports Medicine roundtable on exercise guidelines for cancer survivors. *Medicine and Science in Sports and Exercise, 42,* 1409–1424. doi:10.1249/MSS.0b013e3181e0c112

Seyidova-Khoshknabi, D., Davis, M.P., & Walsh, D. (2011). Review article: A systematic review of cancer-related fatigue measurement questionnaires. *American Journal of Hospice and Palliative Care, 28,* 119–129. doi:10.1177/1049909110381590

CHAPTER **9**

Physical Activity for Cognitive Functioning

Catherine M. Bender, PhD, RN, FAAN

Introduction

Although most individuals with cancer do not experience severe changes in cognitive function, the subtle changes they do experience can interfere with their ability to maintain their usual roles and functions at work, at home, and in the community. This chapter explores the factors (e.g., cancer, treatment) associated with cognitive changes in cancer survivors. The benefits of physical activity and exercise on promoting healthy cognitive functioning are addressed. The FITT principle (see Chapter 4) is applied to assist oncology nurses in creating and evaluating physical activities and exercises appropriate for promoting cognitive function. Oncology nurses can apply this chapter's content to their practice when creating plans of care to support safe physical activity and exercise in cancer survivors. These plans address the activity goals recommended by the National Comprehensive Cancer Network® (NCCN®, 2016) and the American College of Sports Medicine (Schmitz et al., 2010) (see Figure 9-1), as well as the Oncology Nursing Society's *Statement on the Scope and Standards of Oncology Nursing Practice: Generalist and Advanced Practice* (Brant & Wickham, 2013) (see Figure 9-2).

Cognitive Function

Cognitive function is the information handling or information processing component of behavior. Normal cognitive functioning requires the integrated

- Provide assistance with sleep disturbance and fatigue.
- Recommend routine physical activity.
- Encourage patients to engage in general physical activity daily.
- Advise patients to strive for a total of at least 150 minutes of moderate activity or 75 minutes of vigorous activity (or a combination of the two) per week.
- Patients should avoid inactivity.
- Patients should return to normal daily activity as soon as possible following surgery.
- Patients may continue normal daily activities and exercise as much as possible during and after nonsurgical treatments.

Figure 9-1. Clinical Guidelines for Management of Changes in Cognitive Functioning

Note. Based on information from National Comprehensive Cancer Network, 2016.

Standard I. Assessment
- Collect data in the following high-incidence problem areas. These areas may include but are not limited to the following:
  - Protective mechanisms: Neurologic function, including sensory and motor function, level of consciousness, and thought processes
  - Mobility
    * Past and present level of mobility and overall function
    * Risk for decreased mobility
    * Impact of fatigue on mobility
    * Complications related to decreased mobility
  - Survivorship
    * Patient/family understanding of the potential late effects of cancer treatment (e.g., secondary malignancies, organ toxicities, altered fertility, osteoporosis) prior to initiation of therapy
    * Patient/family understanding of the potential persistent or long-term effects associated with cancer treatment (e.g., fatigue, taste changes, cognitive changes, osteoporosis)
    * Patient/family understanding of the need for adherence to long-term follow-up

Standard II. Diagnosis
- Use evidence-based research to formulate the plan of care.

Standard III. Outcome Identification
- Develop expected outcomes for each of the high-incidence problem areas at a level consistent with the patient's physical, psychological, social, and spiritual capacities, cultural background, and value system. The expected outcomes include but are not limited to the following:
  - Mobility: The patient and/or family
    * Incorporate safety and fall prevention strategies in the mobility plan.

Figure 9-2. Standards Applicable to Physical Activity for Promoting Cognitive Functioning

(Continued on next page)

* Describe an appropriate management plan to integrate alteration in mobility into lifestyle.
* Describe optimal levels of activities of daily living at a level consistent with disease state and treatment.
* Identify health services and community resources available for managing changes in mobility.
* Use assistive devices to aid or improve mobility.
* Demonstrate measures to prevent the complications of decreased mobility (e.g., pressure ulcers, pneumonia).

Standard IV. Planning
• Develop the plan of care in collaboration with the patient, family, interdisciplinary cancer care team, and other healthcare professionals when possible.

Standard V. Implementation
• Use evidence-based research to guide implementation of interventions.

Standard VI. Evaluation
• Communicate the patient's response with the interdisciplinary cancer care team and other agencies involved in the healthcare continuum.

Figure 9-2. Standards Applicable to Physical Activity for Promoting Cognitive Functioning (Continued)

Note. From *Statement on the Scope and Standards of Oncology Nursing Practice: Generalist and Advanced Practice,* by J.M. Brant and R. Wickham (Eds.), 2013, Pittsburgh, PA: Oncology Nursing Society. Copyright 2013 by Oncology Nursing Society. Adapted with permission.

action of multiple areas of the brain and is composed of several domains (see Table 9-1) (Matlin, 2005).

The domains of cognitive function are highly integrated with one another such that a problem or impairment in one cognitive domain can have a deleterious effect on other domains. For example, if an individual has a problem maintaining attention when new information is presented, that individual will likely have a problem learning and subsequently remembering that information.

Cognitive function is related to an individual's mood and functional ability (Lezak, Howieson, Loring, Hannay, & Fischer, 2004). Individuals with clinical depression or anxiety are more likely to experience problems with cognitive function. Conversely, those with impairments in cognitive function are more likely to be depressed or anxious. Individuals with cognitive impairments also may experience problems in their ability to function in their usual roles at work, in their family, and in the community. Generally, advancing age is associated with poorer cognitive function, and more years of education and higher general intelligence are related to better cognitive function (Lezak et al., 2004).

Table 9-1. Domains of Cognitive Function

Cognitive Domain	Definition
Attention	Ability to concentrate on a series of stimuli over a period of time
Learning	Acquisition of new information
Memory	Ability to store information for short- or long-term future recall
Psychomotor speed	Speed of performing mental activities with integrated motor responses
Executive function	High-order mental operations that include planning, problem solving, abstract reasoning, and strategy performance
Visuospatial ability	Visual recognition of shapes and forms, organization, and localization in space

Note. Based on information from Lezak, 2004.

Changes in Cognitive Function in Cancer Survivors

Between 30% and 75% of cancer survivors experience changes in cognitive function over the course of their disease and treatment (Jansen, 2013; Wefel, Lenzi, Theriault, Davis, & Meyers, 2004). Changes in cognitive function most commonly involve the domains of attention, concentration, working memory, and executive function (Ahles, Root, & Ryan, 2012). Poorer cognitive function has been documented in survivors with multiple types of cancer and in association with multiple types of treatment, including chemotherapy, immunotherapy, and radiation therapy, particularly when the treatment is delivered directly to the central nervous system (Bender & Thelen, 2013). It is important to keep in mind that although most cancer survivors do not experience severe deterioration in cognitive function or cognitive impairments, they can experience subtler cognitive changes such as difficulty concentrating and recalling recently learned information, making it difficult to function effectively in cognitively challenging environments or situations (Bender & Thelen, 2013).

Recent evidence also indicates that compared to healthy individuals of the same age and education, some cancer survivors have poorer cognitive function before they even begin their cancer treatment, indicating that factors other than therapy are contributing to poorer cognitive function (Ahles et al., 2008; Bender et al., 2013; Hermelink et al., 2015; Wefel et al., 2011). Multiple factors likely contribute to poorer pretherapy cognitive function include the following (Ahles et al., 2008; Bender et al., 2013; Hermelink et al., 2015; Wefel et al., 2011):
• Mood

- Sleep problems
- Symptoms
- Comorbid conditions
- Concomitant medication
- Lingering effects of anesthesia from breast cancer surgery
- Disease-related factors

In addition to the factors that influence cognitive function in healthy individuals, multiple disease- and treatment-related factors may influence changes in cognitive function in cancer survivors.

Cytokine dysregulation: Disease and treatment factors may result in cytokine dysregulation, leading to increased levels of proinflammatory cytokines such as interleukin (IL)-6, IL-1, and C-reactive protein. Higher levels of proinflammatory cytokines are related to poorer cognitive function in patients with cancer (Ahles & Saykin, 2007; Merriman, Von Ah, Miaskowski, & Aouizerat, 2013).

Hormone changes: Changes in levels of hormones such as estrogen may also be related to cognitive decline in cancer survivors. For example, as a consequence of systemic chemotherapy or endocrine therapy, women with breast cancer frequently experience reductions in estrogen levels. Estrogen plays an important role in support of cognitive function, particularly in women, and thus reduced estrogen levels may be related to poorer cognitive function (Ahles & Saykin, 2007; Bender et al., 2006; Merriman et al., 2013).

Genetic variations: Genetic variations also may influence changes in cognitive function in cancer survivors. For example, evidence suggests that variations in genes associated with pathways involved in inflammation, DNA repair, and oxidative stress are related to deteriorations in cognitive function in patients with cancer (Ahles & Saykin, 2007; Merriman et al., 2013).

Cancer-related symptoms: Symptoms experienced by cancer survivors during their disease and treatment, such as fatigue and sleep problems (see Chapters 8 and 11), may be related to poorer cognitive function. Moreover, medications used to manage symptoms, such as antiemetics or narcotic analgesics, also are associated with poorer cognitive function (Bender & Thelen, 2013).

Other factors: Multiple factors increase the risk for developing changes in cognitive function in cancer survivors, as outlined in Figure 9-3.

Potential Benefits of Physical Activity and Exercise for Cognitive Function

Promising evidence suggests that exercise improves cognitive function in healthy adults (Erickson, 2013); however, additional research is needed to confirm these findings (Young, Angevaren, Rusted, & Tabet, 2015). Whether

- Advancing age
- History of neurologic illness or neurotrauma
- History of psychiatric illness such as clinical depression or anxiety disorder
- History of developmental disorders
- History of substance abuse
- Prior cancer treatment
- Cancer therapy delivered directly to the central nervous system (e.g., intrathecal therapy)
- Higher doses of therapy
- Concurrent therapy such as chemoradiation

Figure 9-3. Factors That Increase Risk for Changes in Cognitive Function in Cancer Survivors

Note. Based on information from Hensley et al., 2000.

these same potential cognitive benefits extend to cancer survivors remains unclear, but growing evidence suggests that this may be the case (Mishra, Scherer, Geigle, et al., 2012; Mishra, Scherer, Snyder, et al., 2012).

Two Cochrane reviews examined the effects of exercise on quality of life in patients with cancer during and after completion of treatment (Mishra,

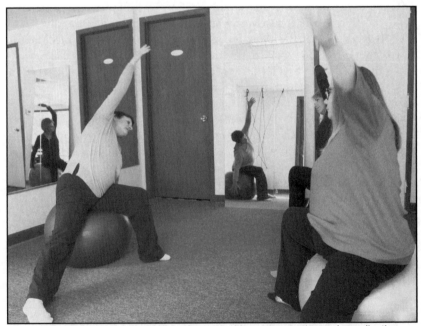

Mindfulness-based exercises, such as those requiring concentration and coordination, improve cognitive function and reduce cognitive complaints in individuals with cancer.

Scherer, Geigle, et al., 2012; Mishra, Scherer, Snyder, et al., 2012). In sub-groups of these two studies, the effects of exercise on self-reported cognitive function in patients with cancer also were explored. No significant effect of exercise on self-reported cognitive function following treatment was identified, but trends were noted in improved self-reported cognitive function with exercise during treatment. It is important to recognize that the authors were not able to examine the frequency, intensity, and duration of exercise in this review. Also, a great deal of heterogeneity existed in the types of exercise examined across the studies, and because cognitive function was not the main focus of the review, no conclusions about the effect of exercise on cognitive function could be drawn. Thus, the potential benefits of exercise for cognitive function in cancer survivors may differ depending on the type of exercise adopted.

Cardiovascular Exercise

Several studies have indicated that four to six months of moderate-intensity aerobic exercise improves executive function, processing speed, and memory in healthy adults (Colcombe & Kramer, 2003; Erickson, 2013; Smith et al., 2010). Changes in these domains of cognitive function frequently are experienced by cancer survivors and therefore may improve with aerobic exercise.

Rogers et al. (2009) found no change in self-reported cognitive function in pre- and postmenopausal women with breast cancer randomized to a 12-week, moderate-intensity walking intervention (N = 20) about three years following diagnosis (Rogers et al., 2009). Knobf, Thompson, Fennie, and Erdos (2014) studied the effects of four to six months of aerobic exercise completed three times each week for up to 45 minutes on symptoms and quality of life in 26 women with breast cancer in a study that used a pretest–post-test design. Outcomes were measured preintervention and then at 16 and 24 weeks following baseline assessment. Although not significant, women reported a trend in reduction in forgetfulness and problems with concentration at 16 weeks (Knobf et al., 2014). After controlling for self-reported exercise behavior, Crowgey et al. (2014) found no difference in cognitive function between women with breast cancer (n = 37) and healthy women (n = 14). Again, these results must be interpreted with great caution because of the small sample size and the use of self-report of exercise. No exercise intervention was instituted in this study.

Resistance Training

Resistance training also may be beneficial for cognitive function in individuals with cancer. In a small sample (N = 17), Baumann et al. (2011) found that women with breast cancer had marginal improvement in short-term verbal memory after 12 weeks of resistance training during chemotherapy compared to a control group of women with breast cancer who did not participate in resistance training during chemotherapy.

Flexibility/Mindfulness Exercise

Research suggests that mindfulness-based exercise improves cognitive function and reduces cognitive complaints in individuals with cancer (Asher & Myers, 2015). Derry et al. (2015) found that breast cancer survivors who participated in a 12-week Hatha yoga intervention had fewer cognitive complaints at three months after the intervention compared to a control group of women with breast cancer who did not participate in Hatha yoga. These results suggest that the benefits of yoga may not be realized immediately (Derry et al., 2015). Oh et al. (2012) reported that 10 weeks of medical Qigong improved self-reported cognitive function in individuals with multiple types of cancer who were completing chemotherapy or had completed chemotherapy compared to a control group of individuals who received usual care during or after chemotherapy. Reid-Arndt, Matsuda, and Cox (2012) reported that women with multiple types of cancer (N = 23) who had completed chemotherapy at least 12 months prior to participation had fewer cognitive complaints and improved memory and attention after completing a 10-week intervention of tai chi.

Oncology Nursing Assessment

Self-Report of Cognitive Functioning

1. Assess cognitive function using self-report. Assessing cancer survivors' self-reported cognitive functioning is one component of an overall health assessment conducted by the oncology nurse. Survivor complaints of changes in cognitive function should prompt the nurse to evaluate for factors that may be contributing to the problem:
   - Type of cancer
   - Treatment protocol
   - Mood
   - Sleep patterns
   - Symptoms (e.g., fatigue)
   - Comorbid conditions
   - Concomitant medications
2. Obtain your oncology center's current assessment scales or questions for cognitive functioning. If none exist, use the information in this chapter to create one. Review the questions you ask cancer survivors about their cognitive functioning.

3. Determine if a referral to a neuropsychologist is needed for cancer survivors with severe or persistent changes in cognitive function (Jansen, 2013).

Self-Report and Physical Activity/Exercise Assessment

1. Assess current physical activity and exercise patterns using measures such as those described in Chapter 4. Use the physical activity and exercise measures endorsed by your oncology center to measure activity. Assessing cancer survivors' current physical activity and exercise program (frequency, intensity, time, and type) will help you understand the levels of physical activity in which survivors are currently engaged.
2. Evaluate the relationship between cancer survivors' physical activity and cognitive function. Assess the frequency, intensity, time, and type of activities. Do the activities require a higher level of cognitive functioning (e.g., activities that require skill, hand-eye coordination, strategy), such as competitive sports? Are the frequency and intensity of activities similar to the evidence presented in this chapter?
3. Evaluate screenings (see Chapter 6) as needed to determine physical readiness for exercise.
4. Determine if a consultation to a physical or occupational therapist is indicated if debilitation is observed.

Oncology Nursing Recommendations for Physical Activity and Exercise to Promote Cognitive Functioning

1. Use any of the interviewing techniques discussed in Chapter 5 to determine cancer survivors' readiness to incorporate physical activity and exercise into their lifestyle.
2. Teach survivors about the potential benefits of physical activity and exercise on improving cognitive functioning. Assure them that an individualized physical activity and exercise plan may promote cognitive function during and after cancer treatment.
3. Use interventions to reduce cancer-related symptom severity and distress, including cognitive impairment, recommended by the Oncology Nursing Society Putting Evidence Into Practice resources (Von Ah et al., 2016)
4. Collaborate with survivors to select physical activities and exercises they enjoy and are able to perform regularly and safely. Use checklists offered by your oncology center or the lists provided in Chapters 1 and 4.
5. Use the FITT principle (see Chapter 4) to collaborate with survivors and create a physical activity and exercise plan. Consider chemotherapy treat-

ment schedules, blood counts, surgery-related restrictions, and other health-related factors when creating a physical activity plan.
6. Calculate the target heart rate zone using the Karvonen formula. Teach survivors how to measure their heart rate and rating of perceived exertion.
7. Provide survivors with a discharge packet for physical activity (see Chapter 8).
8. Ask survivors to bring the tracking program with them on their next visit.

Oncology Nursing Evaluation of Health Outcomes

1. Evaluate cancer survivors' adherence to the recommended physical activity/exercise plan by discussing their self-report outcomes (see Chapter 7).
2. Evaluate these outcomes to the plan adherence and self-reported cognitive function. Note any improvements or worsening in progress.

Application to Oncology Nursing Practice

1. Assessing cognitive functioning is an important component of oncology nursing. Because the changes in cognitive function most commonly experienced by cancer survivors are subtler, most cognitive screening measures are not sensitive to detecting those changes. Comprehensive, multidimensional batteries of neuropsychological measures may detect the subtle changes in cognitive function experienced by most cancer survivors. However, it is not practical and would not be appropriate to administer such batteries on a regular basis in a clinical setting (Bender et al., 2008; Bender, Paraska, Sereika, Ryan, & Berga, 2001).
2. It is important for oncology nurses to be alert to complaints of cognitive problems made by cancer survivors and their caregivers. Such complaints should prompt an assessment of the factors that may be contributing to these problems and ultimately may result in a more comprehensive cognitive assessment by a neuropsychologist.
3. Synthesizing cognitive function assessments with psychosocial and physical readiness for physical activity and exercise allows the oncology nurse to determine a safe approach for creating a doable activity plan. Oncology nurses and cancer survivors can use the FITT principle (see Chapter 4) to create an achievable physical activity plan. Evaluating health outcomes at subsequent visits allows oncology nurses to analyze the effect of the physical activity plan on cognitive function and other health-related outcomes during and after cancer treatment.

Summary

Physical activity and exercise may be effective in mitigating the changes in cognitive function experienced by cancer survivors, but this research is in its early stages. Methodologic concerns, such as small sample sizes and failure to use randomization, exist about much of the research that has been completed to date in this area. Moreover, much of the research that has been done in this area has been in women with breast cancer, and it is not clear whether the results of this research extend to individuals with other types of cancer. Finally, most of the research that has been completed has examined the effects of exercise on self-reported cognitive function. Therefore, it is not known whether exercise improves objectively measured cognition. Additional research is needed to document the potential benefits of exercise for cognitive function in cancer survivors as well as research to determine the frequency, intensity, time, and type of exercises necessary to achieve this benefit.

References

Ahles, T.A., Root, J.C., & Ryan, E.L. (2012). Cancer- and cancer treatment–associated cognitive change: An update on the state of the science. *Journal of Clinical Oncology, 30*, 3675–3686. doi:10.1200/JCO.2012.43.0116

Ahles, T.A., & Saykin, A.J. (2007). Candidate mechanisms for chemotherapy-induced cognitive changes. *Nature Reviews Cancer, 7*, 192–201.

Ahles, T.A., Saykin, A.J., McDonald, B.C., Furstenberg, C.T., Cole, B.F., Hanscom, B.S., ... Kaufman, P.A. (2008). Cognitive function in breast cancer patients prior to adjuvant treatment. *Breast Cancer Research and Treatment, 110*, 143–152. doi:10.1007/s10549-007-9686-5

Asher, A., & Myers, J.S. (2015). The effect of cancer treatment on cognitive function. *Clinical Advances in Hematology and Oncology, 13*(7), 1–10.

Baumann, F.T., Drosselmeyer, N., Leskaroski, A., Knicker, A., Krakowski-Roosen, H., Zopf, E.M., & Bloch, W. (2011). 12-week resistance training with breast cancer patients during chemotherapy: Effects on cognitive abilities. *Breast Care, 6*, 142–143. doi:10.1159/000327505

Bender, C.M., Pacella, M.L., Sereika, S.M., Brufsky, A.M., Vogel, V.G., Rastogi, P., ... Ryan, C.M. (2008). What do perceived cognitive problems reflect? *Journal of Supportive Oncology, 6*, 238–242.

Bender, C.M., Paraska, K.K., Sereika, S.M., Ryan, C.M., & Berga, S.L. (2001). Cognitive function and reproductive hormones in adjuvant therapy for breast cancer: A critical review. *Journal of Pain and Symptom Management, 21*, 407–424. doi:10.1016/S0885-3924(01)00268-8

Bender, C.M., Sereika, S.M., Berga, S.L., Vogel, V.G., Brufsky, A.M., & Ryan, C.M. (2006). Cognitive impairment associated with adjuvant therapy in women with breast cancer. *Psycho-Oncology, 15*, 422–430. doi:10.1002/pon.964

Bender, C.M., Sereika, S.M., Ryan, C.M., Brufsky, A.M., Puhalla, S., & Berga, S.L. (2013). Does lifetime exposure to hormones predict pretreatment cognitive function in women before adjuvant therapy for breast cancer? *Menopause, 20*, 905–913. doi:10.1097/GME.0b013e3182843eff

Bender, C.M., & Thelen, B.D. (2013). Cancer and cognitive changes: The complexity of the problem. *Seminars in Oncology Nursing, 29*, 232–237. doi:10.1016/j.soncn.2013.08.003

Brant, J.M., & Wickham, R. (Eds.). (2013). *Statement on the scope and standards of oncology nursing practice: Generalist and advanced practice.* Pittsburgh, PA: Oncology Nursing Society.

Colcombe, S., & Kramer, A.F. (2003). Fitness effects on the cognitive function of older adults: A meta-analytic study. *Psychological Science, 14*, 125–130. doi:10.1111/1467-9280.t01-1-01430

Crowgey, T., Peters, K.B., Hornsby, W.E., Lane, A., McSherry, F., Herdon, J.E., … Jones, L.W. (2014). Relationship between exercise behavior, cardiorespiratory fitness, and cognitive function in early breast cancer patients treated with doxorubicin-containing chemotherapy: A pilot study. *Applied Physiology, Nutrition, and Metabolism, 39*, 724–729. doi:10.1139/apnm-2013-0380

Derry, H.M., Jaremka, L.M., Bennett, J.M., Peng, J., Andridge, R., Shapiro, C., … Kiecolt-Glaser, J.K. (2015). Yoga and self-reported cognitive problems in breast cancer survivors: A randomized controlled trial. *Psycho-Oncology, 24*, 958–966. doi:10.1002/pon.3707

Erickson, K.I. (2013). Therapeutic effects of exercise on cognitive function. *Journal of the American Geriatrics Society, 61*, 2038–2039. doi:10.1111/jgs.12529

Hensley, M., Peterson, B., Silver, R., Larson, R., Schiffer, C., & Szatrowski, T. (2000). Risk factors for severe neuropsychiatric toxicity in patients receiving interferon alfa-2b and low-dose cytarabine for chronic myelogenous leukemia: Analysis of Cancer and Leukemia Group B 9013. *Journal of Clinical Oncology, 18*, 1301–1308.

Hermelink, K., Voigt, V., Kaste, J., Neufeld, F., Wuerstlein, R., Buhner, M., … Harbeck, N. (2015). Elucidating pretreatment cognitive impairment in breast cancer patients: The impact of cancer-related post-traumatic stress. *Journal of the National Cancer Institute, 107*(7), 1–13. doi:10.1093/jnci/djv099

Jansen, C.E. (2013). Cognitive changes associated with cancer and cancer therapy: Patient assessment and education. *Seminars in Oncology Nursing, 29*, 270–279. doi:10.1016/j.soncn.2013.08.007

Knobf, M.T., Thompson, A.S., Fennie, K., & Erdos, D. (2014). The effect of a community-based exercise intervention on symptoms and quality of life. *Cancer Nursing, 37*, E43–E50. doi:10.1097/NCC.0b013e31828d40e

Lezak, M.D., Howieson, D.B., Loring, D.W., Hannay, H.J., & Fischer, J.S. (2004). *Neuropsychological assessment* (4th ed.). New York, NY: Oxford University Press.

Matlin, M.W. (2005). *Cognition* (6th ed.). New York, NY: John Wiley and Sons.

Merriman, J.D., Von Ah, D., Miaskowski, C., & Aouizerat, B.E. (2013). Proposed mechanisms for cancer- and treatment-related cognitive changes. *Seminars in Oncology Nursing, 29*, 260–269. doi:10.1016/j.soncn.2013.08.006

Mishra, S.I., Scherer, R.W., Geigle, P.M., Berlanstein, D.R., Topaloglu, O., Gotay, C.C., & Snyder, C. (2012). Exercise interventions on health-related quality of life for cancer survivors. *Cochrane Database of Systematic Reviews, 2012*(8). doi:10.1002/14651858.cd007566.pub2

Mishra, S.I., Scherer, R.W., Snyder, C., Geigle, P.M., Berlanstein, D.R., & Topaloglu, O. (2012). Exercise interventions on health-related quality of life for people with cancer during active treatment. *Clinical Otolaryngology, 37*, 390–392. doi:10.1111/coa.12015

National Comprehensive Cancer Network. (2016). *NCCN Clinical Practice Guidelines in Oncology (NCCN Guidelines®): Survivorship* [v.1.2016]. Retrieved from https://www.nccn.org/professionals/physician_gls/pdf/survivorship.pdf

Oh, B., Butow, P.N., Mullan, B.A., Clarke, S.J., Beale, P.J., Pavlakis, N., … Vardy, J. (2012). Effect of medical Qigong on cognitive function, quality of life, and a biomarker of inflammation in cancer patients: A randomized controlled trial. *Supportive Care in Cancer, 20*, 1235–1242. doi:10.1007/s00520-011-1209-6

Reid-Arndt, S.A., Matsuda, S., & Cox, C.R. (2012). Tai Chi effects in neuropsychological, emotional, and physical functioning following cancer treatment: A pilot study. *Complementary Therapies in Clinical Practice, 18*, 26–30. doi:10.1016/j.ctcp.2011.02.005

Rogers, L.Q., Hopkins-Price, P., Vicari, S., Markwell, S., Pamenter, R., Courneya, K.S., … Verhulst, S. (2009). Physical activity and health outcomes three months after completing a physical activity behavior change intervention: Persistent and delayed effects. *Cancer Epidemiology, Biomarkers and Prevention, 18*, 1410–1418. doi:10.1158/1055-9965.EPI-08-1045

Schmitz, K.H., Courneya, K.S., Matthews, C., Demark-Wahnefried, W., Galvão, D.A., Pinto, B.M., … Schwartz, A.L. (2010). American College of Sports Medicine roundtable on exercise guidelines for cancer survivors. *Medicine and Science in Sports and Exercise, 42,* 1409–1426. doi:10.1249/MSS.0b013e3181e0c112

Smith, P.J., Blumenthal, J.A., Hoffman, B.M., Cooper, H., Strauman, T.A., Welsh-Bohmer, K., … Sherwood A. (2010). Aerobic exercise and neurocognitive performance: A meta-analytic review of randomized controlled trials. *Psychosomatic Medicine, 72,* 239–252. doi:10.1097/PSY.0b013e3181d14633

Von Ah, D., Allen, D.H., Jansen, C.E., Merriman, J.D., Myers, J.S., & Wulff, J. (2016). Putting evidence into practice: Cognitive impairment. Retrieved from https://www.ons.org/practice-resources/pep/cognitive-impairment

Wefel, J.S., Lenzi, R., Theriault, R.L., Davis, R.N., & Meyers, C.A. (2004). The cognitive sequelae of standard-dose adjuvant chemotherapy in women with breast carcinoma. *Cancer, 100,* 2292–2299. doi:10.1002/cncr.20272

Wefel, J.S., Vidrine, D.J., Veramonti, T.L., Meyers, C.A., Marani, S.K., Hoekstra, H.J., … Gritz, E.R. (2011). Cognitive impairment in men with testicular cancer prior to adjuvant therapy. *Cancer, 117,* 190–196. doi:10.1002/cncr.25298

Young, J., Angevaren, M., Rusted, J., & Tabet, N. (2015). Aerobic exercise to improve cognitive function in older people without known cognitive impairment. *Cochrane Database of Systematic Reviews, 2015*(4). doi:10.1002/14651858.CD005381.pub4

CHAPTER 10

Physical Activity for Cancer-Related Pain

Justin C. Deskovich, DPT, MPT, OCS, SCS, DAC, CSCS, COMT, FAAOMPT, FMS Cert.

Introduction

All individuals experience physical pain at some point in their lives. Pain serves many valuable functions, such as when to rest, when to seek help, and when an illness or injury is present. Despite these potential positives, there are clearly negative experiences associated with pain. Living in pain or allowing pain to control one's life can lead to disinterest in physical activity and exercise and eventual loss of physical function.

About 50% of cancer survivors experience pain throughout the cancer trajectory (van den Beuken-van Everdingen et al., 2007). van den Beuken-van Everdingen et al. (2007) estimated the prevalence of pain to be 59% among patients in active treatment, 33% among survivors after treatment, and 64% among those with advanced, metastatic, or terminal disease. Furthermore, 75%–90% of cancer survivors will experience life-changing pain from the cancer itself or from cancer-related treatment (Luger, Mach, Sercik, & Mantyh, 2005).

Pain is interrelated with fatigue (see Chapter 8), changes in cognitive function (see Chapter 9), and altered sleep patterns (see Chapter 11). Cancer and pain are associated with deleterious physiologic and psychological effects, ranging from weight gain to decreased quality of life (Goodwin, Bruera, & Stockler, 2014; Mehanna, De Boer, & Morton, 2008; Mystakidou et al., 2007).

Combine the diagnosis of cancer and the presence of pain, and undoubtedly physical activity can decline substantially (Dy, 2010; Fielding, Sanford, & Davis, 2013). Cancer survivors who live with pain are less physically active compared to the general population (Brink-Huis, van Achterberg, & Schoonhoven, 2008; Fallowfield & Jenkins, 2014).

Physical activity and exercise can help cancer survivors cope with or ameliorate their pain. This chapter describes the basic physiology of cancer pain, as well as the effects of physical activity and exercise on cancer pain management. Pain-specific screening and assessment measures applicable to oncology nursing practice are presented. The FITT principle (see Chapter 4) is applied to assist oncology nurses to create and evaluate physical activities and exercises pertinent to pain management. Oncology nurses can incorporate this chapter's content to create individualized plans of care to support safe physical activity as a modality for pain management with cancer survivors. This chapter's content is supported in the Oncology Nursing Society's *Statement on the Scope and Standards of Oncology Nursing Practice: Generalist and Advanced Practice* (Brant & Wickham, 2013) (see Figure 10-1).

Standard I. Assessment
- Collect data in the following high-incidence problem areas. These areas may include but are not limited to the following:
  - Comfort
    * Location, intensity, quality, temporal, and exacerbating and relieving characteristics of discomfort/pain and other deleterious symptoms (e.g., fatigue, nausea, dyspnea, rash, pruritus); nonverbal rating scales for patients who are unable to communicate the presence of symptoms
    * Methods of pain and symptom management, including complementary and alternative modalities and cultural and folk remedies
    * Impact of pain and other distressing symptoms on daily living
  - Mobility
    * Past and present level of mobility and overall function
    * Risk for decreased mobility
    * Impact of fatigue on mobility
    * Complications related to decreased mobility
- Use appropriate evidence-based assessment techniques and instruments in collecting data, including valid and reliable instruments that assess the high-incidence problem areas (e.g., distress thermometer).

Standard II. Diagnosis
- Ensure that nursing diagnoses reflect the patient's actual or potential health problems, including actual or potential alterations in the high-incidence problem areas.

Standard III. Outcome Identification
- Develop expected outcomes for each of the high-incidence problem areas at a level consistent with the patient's physical, psychological, social, and spiritual capacities, cultural background, and value system. The expected outcomes include but are not limited to the following:
  - Comfort
    * Communicate level of distress and changes in comfort level using an agreed-upon pain/symptom rating scale.

Figure 10-1. Standards Applicable to Physical Activity for Managing Cancer-Related Pain

---

(Continued on next page)

* Describe the source of the distress or discomfort, treatment measures, and expected outcomes.
* Identify measures to enhance physical, psychological, social, spiritual, cultural, and environmental factors that increase comfort and promote the continuance of valued activities and relationships.
* Describe appropriate interventions for potential or predictable problems, such as pain, fatigue, dyspnea, sleep pattern disturbances, nausea, vomiting, and pruritus.
* Participate in self-care for symptom management.
* Contact an appropriate cancer care team member when symptom control is ineffective.
 – Mobility
    * Describe an appropriate management plan to integrate alteration in mobility into lifestyle.
    * Describe optimal levels of activities of daily living at a level consistent with disease state and treatment.
    * Identify health services and community resources available for managing changes in mobility.
    * Use assistive devices to aid or improve mobility.
    * Demonstrate measures to prevent the complications of decreased mobility (e.g., pressure ulcers, pneumonia).

Standard IV. Planning
• Develop the plan of care in collaboration with the patient, family, interdisciplinary cancer care team, and other healthcare professionals when possible.

Standard V. Implementation
• Use evidence-based research to guide implementation of interventions.

Standard VI. Evaluation
• Communicate the patient's response with the interdisciplinary cancer care team and other agencies involved in the healthcare continuum.

Figure 10-1. Standards Applicable to Physical Activity for Managing Cancer-Related Pain *(Continued)*

Note. From *Statement on the Scope and Standards of Oncology Nursing Practice: Generalist and Advanced Practice,* by J.M. Brant and R. Wickham (Eds.), 2013, Pittsburgh, PA: Oncology Nursing Society. Copyright 2013 by Oncology Nursing Society. Adapted with permission.

Cancer-Related Pain

The International Association for the Study of Pain (IASP) defines pain as "an unpleasant sensory and emotional experience associated with actual or potential tissue damage" (IASP, 2014, para. 1). Pain corresponds to a sensory and emotional experience that must be detected by the brain. Ultimately, the brain determines if "danger" is present. Pain often is not evident in malignancies, and by the time the individual seeks care, the cancer may have metastasized. In general, pain involves the brain and nervous system and is different for every individual (Louw, 2013).

Acute and Chronic Cancer-Related Pain

Cancer survivors may experience both acute and chronic pain. Acute pain functions as a warning system to alert individuals that something is wrong or potentially wrong with their body. Once the source of acute cancer pain is discovered, treated appropriately, and healed, the pain usually resolves rather quickly (Briggs, 2010). Unless the patient experiences cancer- or treatment-related side effects (e.g., pathologic fracture, bowel obstruction, hemorrhage, compressed nerve-sensitive structures), cancer rarely causes acute pain. Most acute cancer-related pain is caused by diagnostic procedures, surgical procedures, infection, or treatment. Table 10-1 lists common causes of acute pain in cancer survivors.

Chronic pain does not serve as a pain that is required for survival; chronic pain occurring for months, years, or a lifetime serves no valuable function. Chronic pain lasts longer than the expected healing time and may have no cause whatsoever (Briggs, 2010). Such pain debilitates people and costs billions of dollars in health-related expenses (Gaskin & Richard, 2012). Thus, chronic pain in cancer survivors can be subclassified as chronic malignant pain or chronic nonmalignant pain. Table 10-2 lists common causes of chronic pain in cancer survivors.

Table 10-1. Common Causes of Acute Pain in Cancer Survivors

Type of Pain	Examples
Postoperative pain	Acute inflammatory response, wound pain, neuritis, catheter pain, drain tube pain, hematoma
Diagnostic procedural pain	Biopsies, spinal taps, blood draws, other punctures
Pain associated with chemotherapy	Mucositis, colony-stimulating factor–related pain, infusion-related pain, venous spasm, chemical phlebitis, chemotherapy-induced peripheral neuropathy
Pain associated with radiation therapy	Mucositis, proctitis, enteritis, neuritis, cystitis, pancreatitis, radiation burns
Pain associated with immunotherapy	Myalgia from interferon or interleukin therapy, ostealgia from interferon or interleukin therapy
Pain associated with hormonal therapy	Headaches, arthralgia, estrogen therapy, mastalgia, prostatitis, androgen therapy
Pain associated with infection	Abscess, acute herpetic neuralgia, wound infection
Acute pain associated with tumors	Plexopathy, myelopathy, radiculopathy, pathologic fractures, acute obstruction, meningitis, deep vein thrombosis

Note. Based on information from Chapman, 2011.

Table 10-2. Common Causes of Chronic Pain in Cancer Survivors

Type of Pain	Examples
Treatment-related chronic pain	Postsurgical phantom pain, postsurgical neuropathy, postsurgical radiculopathy, chemotherapy-induced peripheral neuropathy, radiation-induced plexopathy, radiation myelopathy, radiation-induced neuroma, hormone treatment–related pain with prostate and breast cancer (i.e., gynecomastia)
Neuropathic-related pain	Tumor-induced peripheral neuropathy, tumor-induced radiculopathy, tumor-induced myelopathy, tumor-induced plexopathy
Ostealgia-related pain	Primary osteosarcoma, osteologic metastasis, myelopathy from metastasis, osteonecrosis
Visceral-related pain	Pancreatic malignancy, hepatic malignancy, ovarian malignancy, colorectal malignancy, chronic intestinal obstruction, chronic ureter obstruction, hepatic distension
Phantom pain	Postmastectomy, postcolectomy, postsurgical removal of an organ, limb, or part of body

Cancer survivors experiencing acute or chronic pain have greater anxiety and depression in relation to function compared to survivors who do not have cancer-related pain (Chen, Chang, & Yeh, 2000). Identifying cognitive-affective mechanisms in cancer pain may help oncology nurses incorporate cognitive behavioral therapy, including patient education, pain coping strategies, and relaxation techniques (e.g., diaphragmatic breathing, distraction), to encourage patient acceptance of current medical status. Physical activity and exercise can be beneficial as a safe intervention for these health conditions.

Benefits of Physical Activity and Exercise on Cancer-Related Pain

Physical activity and exercise can be beneficial to manage cancer pain as well as boost energy levels, decrease fatigue (see Chapter 8), relieve stress, improve flexibility, and strengthen muscles (American Cancer Society, 2014). The National Comprehensive Cancer Network® (NCCN®) guidelines note that pain is likely to be relieved, or function improved, with modalities such as bed, bath, and walking supports; positioning instruction; instruction in therapeutic and conditioning exercise; and energy conservation and pacing of activities (NCCN, 2016a). The NCCN guidelines also recommend physical activity and exercise for specific adult cancer-related pain conditions (see Figure

- Patients should obtain medical clearance and referral, if needed, before beginning a physical activity program.
- Recommend routine physical activity.
- Tailor physical activities to survivors' abilities and preferences.
- Advise patients to strive for a total of at least 150 minutes of moderate activity or 75 minutes of vigorous activity (or a combination of the two) per week.
- Include endurance (cardiovascular), strength, and stretching modalities.
- Patients should avoid inactivity.
- Patients should return to normal daily activity as soon as possible following surgery.
- Patients may continue normal daily activities and exercise as much as possible during and after nonsurgical treatments.

Figure 10-2. Clinical Guidelines for Promoting a Healthy Lifestyle

Note. Based on information from National Comprehensive Cancer Network, 2016b.

10-2) (NCCN, 2016b). Consultation with a physical or occupational therapist or physical medicine specialist is recommended to ensure appropriate exercise prescription and proper assistive devices based on the cancer pain syndrome.

The research conducted on the effects of physical activity and exercise on cancer-related pain shows promise in helping cancer survivors cope with or diminish pain. Most of this research includes pain as a component of overall

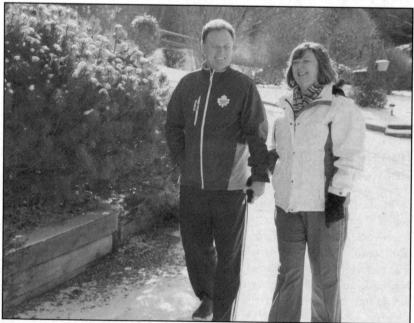

Walking outdoors is an activity that may ameliorate pain and discomfort.

quality of life. Although pain measurement scales vary across the studies, the outcomes of physical activity and exercise programs demonstrate decreases in pain among study participants.

Cardiovascular/Aerobic Exercise

Alfano et al. (2007) conducted a study with 545 breast cancer survivors to determine the patient relationship with physical activity, occurrence of physical symptoms, and health-related quality of life. Interviews were conducted either in person or via mail starting 29 and 39 months following cancer diagnosis. Pain and other quality-of-life factors were measured. Increased physical activity following cancer diagnosis was related to less pain, less fatigue, and better physical functioning. No differences were observed between Hispanic and non-Hispanic women in outcome measures. Of interest was that decreases in fatigue and bodily pain were found with moderate and vigorous sports and recreational physical activity but not household activity.

Physical Exercise During Adjuvant Chemotherapy Effectiveness Study (PACES), a multisite study, evaluated the effects of a low-intensity, home-based physical activity program called Onco-Move and a moderate- to high-intensity, supervised resistance and aerobic exercise program called OnTrack (van Waart et al., 2015). Onco-Move, an individualized, self-managed physical activity program, incorporated components of the transtheoretical model of behavior change (see Chapter 5). Written information was provided that matched cancer survivors' stage of preparedness to exercise and included an activity diary that was discussed at each chemotherapy cycle. Nurses who were trained in the behavior change technique encouraged participants to be physically active for at least 30 minutes per day for five days a week, with an intensity level of 12–14 (out of 20) on the Borg rating scale (see Chapters 4 and 7). OnTrack was described as a strength and resistance exercise program. Usual care, the third group in the study, lacked a specific exercise program for participants. The outcome measures were physical fitness parameters, fatigue, quality of life (including pain), and chemotherapy completion rates.

In this study, 230 breast cancer survivors were randomized to Onco-Move, OnTrack, or usual care. Compared with the usual care group, the Onco-Move and OnTrack participants had improvements in physical functioning, including cardiorespiratory fitness, and less pain. Compared to the Onco-Move and usual care groups, the OnTrack group displayed improved outcomes in muscle strength and fatigue. Both exercise programs resulted in improved pain outcomes for women with breast cancer undergoing chemotherapy (VanWaart et al., 2015).

Strength/Resistance Exercise

The PACES study utilized a supervised combined resistance and aerobic exercise program (OnTrack) as part of its study. OnTrack was a moderate- to high-intensity, combined resistance and aerobic exercise program that was supervised by physical therapists. OnTrack participants attended two sessions per week. Six large muscle groups were trained for 20 minutes per session, with two series of eight reps at 80% of the one-repetition maximum, or 1RM (see Chapter 4). Each session incorporated 30 minutes of aerobic exercise. The intensity was adjusted using the Borg rating scale. Participants were encouraged to be physically active five days each week for 30 minutes per session and to keep an activity diary. OnTrack participants reported less pain compared to the Onco-Move and usual care groups, as well as improvements in muscular strength and endurance.

Flexibility Exercise

Research shows that yoga as a physical activity modality demonstrates an improvement in pain. The effect of Hatha yoga on quality of life and psychosocial functioning was studied in 24 breast cancer survivors over a 12-week period. Pre- and postassessments showed improvements in quality-of-life indicators, including bodily pain (mean change, +4.4; $p = 0.024$) (Speed-Andrews, Stevinson, Belanger, Mirus, & Courneya, 2010). In a study comparing the effects of yoga and exercise on quality of life in cancer survivors aged 65–70 years, Yagli and Ulger (2015) found that both the yoga and exercise groups had improved quality-of-life parameters, including improvements in fatigue, sleep quality, and pain (measured with visual analog scales) ($p < 0.05$). Sudarshan et al. (2013) studied the impact of a 12-week yoga therapy program on anxiety, depression, and physical health in breast cancer survivors (42.8% with total mastectomy and 15.4% with breast reconstruction). Pain was measured with the Dallas Pain Questionnaire. Improvements in pain were noted at the completion of the study.

These exemplars of research demonstrate that physical activity and exercise programs reduce pain in program participants. Most of the studies had small sample sizes, were conducted in breast cancer survivors, and utilized various pain measurement scales; future studies should include other types of cancer, consistent pain measurements, and larger sample sizes.

Oncology Nursing Assessment

Assessing for the presence of acute and chronic pain is an essential component of oncology nursing practice throughout treatment and follow-up visits. Pain assessment measures should be age and culturally appropriate. Assessment measures used in special populations (e.g., visual impairment, dementia) should be available. Asking family members and caregivers about the cancer survivor's pain experience adds another dimension of assessment and creates an opportunity to learn about physical activity patterns for the survivor and family.

Self-Report and Pain Assessment

1. Assess for pain using valid and reliable self-report measures. One self-report is the short-form McGill Pain Questionnaire, which is a valid measure of pain in both younger and older cancer survivors (Gauthier et al., 2014; Melzack, 1975). A numeric pain rating scale is another option, as are pediatric-specific scales (e.g., Wong-Baker FACES pain rating scale; for a modified version of the Wong-Baker pain rating scale, see Figure 10-3). The WILDA approach is another method for pain assessment (see Figure 10-4).

2. Obtain your oncology center's current pain assessment scales. Review the questions cancer survivors are asked about the presence of pain, and compare your center's practice with the assessments listed in this chapter.

3. Assess for pain using subjective questions (see Figure 10-5).

4. Assess for pain using objective criteria by observing the cancer survivor move and ambulate. Observations may include the following:
   - Gait: Favoring one side; limping; uneven gait sequence even when using an assistive device such as a cane, walker, or crutches; and avoiding or limiting movement
   - Carrying and holding objects: Using one hand or one arm only, favoring one arm
   - Self-pain relief: Rubbing a body area; splinting a body area; wearing a brace, heat pack, or ice pack
   - Verbal response to movement: Light cry, verbal pain indicators (e.g., "Ouch!")
   - Facial expressions: Grimacing, crying, lip biting or pursing, wincing, uneven breathing patterns or holding breath during movement

5. Review the cancer survivor's medication regimen for pharmacologic agents used to treat pain, including prescription medications, over-the-counter medications, and supplements.

6. Determine if a referral for pain services is needed based on self-assessment and nursing assessment.

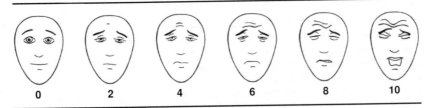

| 0 | 2 | 4 | 6 | 8 | 10 |

Figure 10-3. Faces Scale and Numeric Pain Rating

Note. Copyright 2001 by International Association for the Study of Pain. Retrieved from http://www.iasp-pain.org/Education/Content.aspx?ItemNumber=1519&navItemNumber=577. Used with permission.

Words to describe pain: What does your pain feel like? What words would you use to describe your pain? Have patient describe; avoid providing words to patient.

☐aching   ☐throbbing   ☐shooting   ☐stabbing

☐gnawing   ☐sharp   ☐tender   ☐burning

☐exhausting   ☐penetrating   ☐nagging   ☐pressure

☐numb   ☐miserable   ☐unbearable   ☐dull

☐radiating   ☐tingling   ☐crampy   ☐deep

Intensity of the pain: On a scale of 0 to 10, with 0 being no pain at all and 10 being the worst pain you can imagine, what is your pain now? Has its intensity changed? What has it been in the last 24 hours?

Location of the pain: Where is your pain? Is there more than one site?

Duration of the pain: When did your pain start? How often does it occur? Is the pain always there? Does the pain come and go? (Breakthrough pain)

Aggravating/alleviating factors: What makes your pain better? What makes your pain worse?

Additional Areas for Assessment
Vital signs, past medication history, knowledge of pain management, and use of non-pharmacologic pain relief techniques

How does the pain affect physical and social functioning?

☐sleep   ☐energy   ☐relationships   ☐appetite   ☐activity   ☐mood

Is patient experiencing pain medication side effects?

☐constipation   ☐sedation   ☐itching   ☐nausea   ☐urinary retention

☐confusion   ☐vomiting   ☐dry mouth   ☐hallucinations

Figure 10-4. WILDA Pain Assessment Guide

Note. Copyright 2013 by Regina Fink, RN, PhD, FAAN, AOCN®, University of Colorado Health. Used with permission.

Duration: When did your pain first start?
Location: Where is your pain located?
Intensity: When is your pain at best and at worst?
Quality: What does your pain feel like?
Function: How does your pain affect your daily activities?
Time of Day: At what time is your pain the worst?
Aggravating Factors: What makes your pain worse?
Relieving Factors: What makes your pain better?

Figure 10-5. Subjective Pain Assessment

Self-Report and Physical Activity/Exercise Assessment

Assess current physical activity and exercise patterns using measures such as those described in Chapters 4 and 6. Use the physical activity and exercise measures endorsed by your oncology center to measure activity. Assessing cancer survivors' current physical activity and exercise program (frequency, intensity, time, and type) will help you understand the level of physical activity in which survivors are currently engaged.

1. Evaluate the relationship between the cancer survivor's physical activity and pain. Assess the frequency, intensity, time, and type of activities. Are the types of activities performed creating pain or discomfort? Is there a pattern between activities and the onset, duration, or amelioration of pain?
2. Use screenings as needed to determine physical readiness for exercise (see Chapter 7).
3. Determine if a consultation with a physical or occupational therapist or pain service is indicated if debilitation is observed or if pain is experienced with physical activity or exercise.

Oncology Nursing Recommendations for Physical Activity and Exercise to Manage Cancer-Related Pain

1. Use any of the interviewing techniques discussed in Chapter 5 to determine cancer survivors' readiness to incorporate physical activity and exercise into their lifestyle.
2. Teach survivors about the potential benefits of physical activity and exercise on cancer-related pain. Use the evidence presented in this chapter to create a patient education sheet. Use the education materials provided by your oncology center. Assure survivors that an individualized physical activity and exercise plan can help to relieve cancer-related pain during and after cancer treatment.
3. Teach survivors about cancer-related pain. Learning about pain decreases the threat value of pain (Moseley, 2003). The lower the threat value of pain, the more likely survivors are to participate in physical activity and exercise. Understanding pain science and exercise improves physical health, decreases pain, and improves quality of life in chronic pain (Moseley, 2002, 2003).
4. Collaborate with survivors to select physical activities and exercises they enjoy and are able to perform regularly and safely. Use checklists offered by your oncology center or the lists provided in Chapters 1 and 4.
5. Use the FITT principle (see Chapter 4) to collaborate with survivors and create a physical activity and exercise plan.
6. Consider chemotherapy treatment schedules, blood counts, surgery-related restrictions, and other health-related factors when creating a physical activity plan (see Chapter 7).

7. Match physical activity and exercise plans to the subjective and objective pain assessments. Recommend physical activities and exercises that are known to help with pain management. If survivors receive proper instruction and believe exercise will decrease their pain and improve their endurance, strength, and overall quality of life, they may be more likely to engage in physical activities and exercises. Calculate the target heart rate zone and teach cancer survivors how to measure their heart rate and rating of perceived exertion (see Chapters 6 and 7).

8. Provide a discharge packet for physical activity to manage cancer-related pain that includes the following (see Chapter 8):
   • Self-report pain questionnaire
   • Pain diary (see Figure 10-6)

9. Set short-term (daily or weekly) and long-term (monthly) goals with survivors and their families for physical activity and exercise to gradually reach 150 minutes of aerobic activity per week (Jankowski & Matthews, 2011).

10. Educate cancer survivors on the difference between muscle soreness due to physical activity and pain due to cancer.

11. Advise survivors to select a method for tracking physical activity and pain onset and duration. Ask survivors to bring the tracking program with them on their next visit.

Day	Date	At what time today did you experience your worst pain?	What caused your pain?	What did you do to treat or alleviate your pain?
Monday				
Tuesday				
Wednesday				
Thursday				
Friday				
Saturday				
Sunday				

Figure 10-6. Pain Diary

12. Recommend support systems, such as a walking partner or group, and resources, including indoor walking facilities, to initiate and maintain an active physical activity and exercise plan.

Oncology Nursing Evaluation of Health Outcomes

1. Evaluate cancer survivors' adherence to the recommended physical activity and/or exercise plan by discussing their self-report outcomes. Note any improvements in or worsening of pain experiences.
2. Ask cancer survivors about their experiences with their physical activity and exercise plan and their pain experience.
3. Revise physical activity and exercise plans as needed. Adjust the frequency, intensity, time, and type of activities to meet the survivor's needs for adequate pain management.
4. Follow up with referrals for pain services and physical or occupational therapy as required by your oncology center.

Application to Oncology Nursing Practice

1. Pain assessment is an important component of oncology nursing. Synthesizing self-reported pain assessments with psychosocial and physical readiness for physical activity and exercise allows oncology nurses to determine a safe approach for creating feasible activity plans to augment pain management and promote comfort.
2. Oncology nurses and cancer survivors can use the FITT principle to create an achievable physical activity plan.
3. Evaluating health outcomes at subsequent visits allows oncology nurses to analyze the effect of the physical activity plan on pain and other health-related outcomes during and after cancer treatment.

Summary

Cancer survivors who experience pain can benefit from physical activity and exercise. Physical activity and exercise programs should prove individualized and comprehensive according to the survivor's current fitness level, health history, type of cancer, cancer treatments, adverse effects of treatments, and whether the survivor is undergoing or has completed treatments (Jankowski & Matthews, 2011). Careful attention to physical activity and exercise science principles, in combination with patient education about pain, can improve adherence to physical activity and exercise programming.

Case Study

N.F. is a 39-year-old woman who was diagnosed with an aggressive form of breast cancer six weeks ago. N.F. has minimal and declining social interaction with friends. She works a high-stress job as a secretary, where she spends a significant amount of time on the computer and phone. Prior to diagnosis, N.F. walked three to five times per week with friends for 45 minutes to lose weight. She experiences dull, aching low back pain on her right side with prolonged sitting at work and with prolonged walking (greater than 20 minutes for both activities). Her pain becomes sharp when she bends, lifts, twists, and squats. Although the pain wakes her up, N.F. is able to return to sleep with a change in position. She worries her cancer has spread to her back and is afraid to exercise because her pain ranges from 2/10 to 10/10. Her goals are to eliminate her low back pain, return to work and leisure activities without limitations of pain, and begin an exercise program (see Figure 10-7).

Relevant Laboratory Values
• All within normal limits

Medical History
• Depression
• Anxiety
• Low back pain
• Osteoarthritis in bilateral knees
• Plantar fasciitis
• Hypothyroidism
• Family history of cancer
• Mastectomy

Medications
• Acetaminophen PRN for joint pain
• Fluvoxamine

Height/weight	• Height: 5'5" • Weight: 175 lbs • BMI: 29 • Overweight
Vitals	• Blood pressure: 115/72 mm Hg • Resting heart rate: 83 bpm • Respiratory rate: 20 breaths per minute • Temperature: 98.6°F (37°C)
Cardiopulmonary	• Normal lung sounds bilaterally • Normal cardiovascular examination
Other	• All myotomes and dermatomes within normal limits bilaterally • Deep tendon reflex, 2/4 bilateral patellar, medial hamstrings, and Achilles • Negative clonus

Figure 10-7. Additional Patient Information

BMI—body mass index; bpm—beats per minute

Physical Activity Management Plan

- Educate patient about the following:
  - Ergonomics
  - Characteristics of mechanical low back pain
  - Realistic expectations for recovery
  - Neuroscience of pain
- Encourage patient to resume walking with friends within tolerance.
- Advise patient to begin yoga and/or meditation at home.
- Refer patient to physical therapy for evaluation of low back pain and education on body mechanics in addition to a supervised exercise program to improve her function and return to work and leisure activities.
- Determine target training heart rate (HR) using the Karvonen formula:
  1. Maximum HR (MHR) = 220 (constant) − 39 (patient's age) = 181 beats per minute (bpm)
  2. HR reserve = 181 (MHR) − 83 (resting HR [RHR]) = 98 bpm
  3. Initial desired exercise intensity = light to moderate (40%–60% target heart rate)
  4. Target training HR = 98 (HR reserve) × 0.40 (desired intensity) + 83 (RHR) = 122 bpm
  5. Target training HR = 98 (HR reserve) × 0.60 (desired intensity) + 83 (RHR) = 142 bpm

---

Sample Exercise Prescription

Exercise Type	Frequency	Intensity	Time	Type
Strength and flexibility	2 times per week	Low load to point of resistance and ability to maintain proper position	30 minutes of yoga and 5 minutes seated meditation	Yoga and daily meditation (focus on strength and hip mobility)
Cardiovascular	5 times per week	40%–60% maximum heart rate, rating of perceived exertion of 4/10, or able to talk while moving (see Table 4-3 in Chapter 4)	30–45 minutes	Walking

(Continued on next page)

Sample Exercise Prescription *(Continued)*				
Exercise Type	Frequency	Intensity	Time	Type
Resistance training*	3 times per week	65% of one-repetition maximum (see Chapter 4)	8–10 exercises addressing major muscle groups	Weight lifting under trainer supervision

* Plan to have patient rest from upper extremity resistance training during tissue healing from surgical intervention. This may include modifications to beginner yoga practice in early stages.

Follow-Up

Six months following completion of treatment, Nancy reports a weight loss of six pounds. She also reports an increase in energy; she no longer wakes up from low back pain. Nancy is currently independent in an exercise program and knows how to modify her workout routine if she experiences pain symptoms.

References

Alfano, C.M., Smith, A.W., Irwin, M.L., Bowen, D.J., Sorensen, B., Reeve, B.B., … McTiernan, A. (2007). Physical activity, long-term symptoms, and physical health-related quality of life among breast cancer survivors: A prospective analysis. *Journal of Cancer Survivorship, 1,* 116–128. doi:10.1007/s11764-007-0014-1

American Cancer Society. (2014). Physical activity and the cancer patient. Retrieved from http://www.cancer.org/treatment/survivorshipduringandaftertreatment/stayingactive/physical-activity-and-the-cancer-patient

Brant, J.M., & Wickham, R. (Eds.). (2013). *Statement on the scope and standards of oncology nursing practice: Generalist and advanced practice.* Pittsburgh, PA: Oncology Nursing Society.

Briggs, E. (2010). Understanding the experience and physiology of pain. *Nursing Standard, 3,* 35–39. doi:10.7748/ns2010.09.25.3.35.c7989

Brink-Huis, A., van Achterberg, T., & Schoonhoven, L. (2008). Pain management: A review of organisation models with integrated processes for the management of pain in adult cancer patients. *Journal of Clinical Nursing, 17,* 1986–2000. doi:10.1111/j.1365-2702.2007.02228.x

Chapman, S. (2011). Assessment and management of patients with cancer pain. *Cancer Nursing Practice, 10*(10), 28–36. doi:10.7748/cnp2011.12.10.10.28.c8867

Chen, M.L., Chang, H.K., & Yeh, C.H. (2000). Anxiety and depression in Taiwanese cancer patients with and without pain. *Journal of Advanced Nursing, 32,* 944–951.

Dy, S.M. (2010). Evidence-based approaches to pain in advanced cancer. *Cancer Journal, 16,* 500–506. doi:10.1097/PPO.0b013e3181f45853

Fallowfield, L., & Jenkins, V. (2014). Psychosocial/survivorship issues in breast cancer: Are we doing better? *Journal of the National Cancer Institute, 107,* 335. doi:10.1093/jnci/dju335

Fielding, F., Sanford, T.M., & Davis, M.P. (2013). Achieving effective control in cancer pain: A review of current guidelines. *International Journal of Palliative Nursing, 19,* 584–591. doi:10.12968/ijpn.2013.19.12.584

Gaskin, D.J., & Richard, P. (2012). The economic costs of pain in the United States. *Journal of Pain, 13,* 715–724. doi:10.1016/j.jpain.2012.03.009

Gauthier, L.R., Young, A., Dworkin, R.H., Rodin, G., Zimmermann, C., Warr, D., ... Gagliese, L. (2014). Validation of the short-form McGill Pain Questionnaire-2 in younger and older people with cancer pain. *Journal of Pain, 15,* 756–770. doi:10.1016/j.jpain.2014.04.004

Goodwin, P.J., Bruera, E., & Stockler, M. (2014). Pain in patients with cancer. *Journal of Clinical Oncology, 32,* 1637–1639. doi:10.1200/JCO.2014.55.3818

International Association for the Study of Pain. (2014). IASP taxonomy. Retrieved from http://www.iasp-pain.org/Taxonomy

Jankowski, C.M., & Matthews, E.E. (2011). Exercise guidelines for adults with cancer: A vital role in survivorship. *Clinical Journal of Oncology Nursing, 15,* 683–686. doi:10.1188/11.CJON .683-686

Louw, A. (2013). *Why do I hurt? A patient book about the neuroscience of pain.* Minneapolis, MN: Orthopedic Physical Therapy Products.

Luger, N.M., Mach, D.B., Sevcik, M.A., & Mantyh, P.W. (2005). Bone cancer pain: From model to mechanism to therapy. *Journal of Pain and Symptom Management, 29,* S32–S46. doi:10.1016/j.jpainsymman.2005.01.008

Mehanna, H.M., De Boer, M.F., & Morton, R.P. (2008). The association of psycho-social factors and survival in head and neck cancer. *Clinical Otolaryngology, 33,* 83–89. doi:10.1111/j.1749 -4486.2008.01666.x

Melzack, R. (1975). The McGill Pain Questionnaire: Major properties and scoring methods. *Pain, 1,* 277–299. doi:10.1016/0304-3959(75)90044-5

Moseley, G.L. (2002). Combined physiotherapy and education is efficacious for chronic low back pain. *Australian Journal of Physiotherapy, 48,* 297–302. doi:10.1016/S0004-9514(14)60169-0

Moseley, G.L. (2003). Joining forces—Combining cognition–targeted motor control training with group or individual pain physiology education: A successful treatment for chronic low back pain. *Journal of Manual and Manipulative Therapy, 11,* 88–94. doi:10.1179/106698103790826383

Mystakidou, K., Tsilika, E., Parpa, E., Pathiaki, M., Patiraki, E., Galanos, A., & Vlahos, L. (2007). Exploring the relationships between depression, hopelessness, cognitive status, pain, and spirituality in patients with advanced cancer. *Archives of Psychiatric Nursing, 21,* 150–161. doi:10.1016/j.apnu.2007.02.002

National Comprehensive Cancer Network. (2016a). *NCCN Clinical Practice Guidelines in Oncology (NCCN Guidelines®): Adult cancer pain* [v.2.2016]. Retrieved from https://www.nccn.org/professionals/physician_gls/pdf/pain.pdf

National Comprehensive Cancer Network. (2016b). *NCCN Clinical Practice Guidelines in Oncology (NCCN Guidelines®): Survivorship* [v.1.2016]. Retrieved from https://www.nccn.org/professionals/physician_gls/pdf/survivorship.pdf

Rehabilitation Measures Database. (1994). Oswestry Disability Index. Retrieved from http://www.rehabmeasures.org/Lists/RehabMeasures/DispForm.aspx?ID=1114

Speed-Andrews, A.E., Stevinson, C., Belanger, L.J., Mirus, J.J., & Courneya, K.S. (2010). Pilot evaluation of an Iyengar yoga program for breast cancer survivors. *Cancer Nursing, 33,* 369–381. doi:10.1097/NCC.0b013e3181cfb55a

Sudarshan, M., Petrucci, A., Dumitra, S., Duplisea, J., Wexler, S., & Meterissian, S. (2013). Yoga therapy for breast cancer patients: A prospective cohort study. *Complementary Therapies in Clinical Practice, 19,* 227–229. doi:10.1016/j.ctcp.2013.06.004

van den Beuken-van Everdingen, M.H., de Rijke, J.M., Kessels, A.G., Schouten, H.C., van Kleef, M., & Patijn, J. (2007). Prevalence of pain in patients with cancer: A systematic review of the past 40 years. *Annals of Oncology, 18,* 1437–1449.

van Waart, H., Stuiver, M.M., van Harten, W.H., Geleijn, E., Kieffer, J.M., Buffart, L.M., ... Aaronson, N.K. (2015). Effect of low-intensity physical activity and moderate-to high-intensity physical exercise during adjuvant chemotherapy on physical fitness, fatigue, and chemotherapy completion rates: Results of the PACES randomized clinical trial. *Journal of Clinical Oncology, 33,* 1918–1927. doi:10.1200/JCO.2014.59.1081

Yagli, N., & Ulger, O. (2015). The effects of yoga on the quality of life and depression in elderly breast cancer patients. *Complementary Therapies in Clinical Practice, 21,* 7–10. doi:10.1016/j. ctcp.2015.01.002

CHAPTER 11

Physical Activity for Promoting Sleep

Ann M. Berger, PhD, APRN, AOCNS®, FAAN, and Ellyn E. Matthews, PhD, RN, AOCNS®, CBSM, FAAN

Introduction

Many people, including those living with cancer, have difficulty falling and staying asleep several nights per week. Lack of sleep results in fatigue and daytime sleepiness, which may prevent individuals from carrying out their activities of daily living or participating in physical activity.

Compared with fatigue, pain, and cognitive functioning, little attention is paid to the relationship between sleep and physical activity among cancer survivors. This chapter describes the basic tenets of sleep, as well as the benefits of physical activity and exercise on sleep for cancer survivors. Screening and assessment measures related to sleep that are applicable to oncology nursing practice are presented. The FITT principle (see Chapter 4) is applied to assist oncology nurses in creating and evaluating physical activities pertinent to promoting restorative sleep (American Council on Exercise, 2003). Oncology nurses can incorporate this chapter's content to create individualized plans of care to promote physical activities that support restful sleep in cancer survivors. These plans address the activity goals recommended by the National Comprehensive Cancer Network® (NCCN®) guidelines (NCCN, 2015) and the American College of Sports Medicine (Schmitz et al., 2010). This chapter's content is supported in the Oncology Nursing Society's *Statement on the Scope and Standards of Oncology Nursing Practice: Generalist and Advanced Practice* (Brant & Wickham, 2013) (see Figure 11-1).

Standard I. Assessment
- Collect data in the following high-incidence problem areas. These areas may include but are not limited to the following:
  - Health promotion
    * Environmental risk factors
    * Personal risk factors, including genetic factors
    * Health promotion and disease prevention practices
    * Early detection practices
    * Cultural and social factors
  - Mobility
    * Past and present level of mobility and overall function
    * Risk for decreased mobility
    * Impact of fatigue on mobility
    * Complications related to decreased mobility
  - Survivorship: Patient/family understanding of the potential persistent or long-term effects associated with cancer treatment (e.g., fatigue, taste changes, cognitive changes, osteoporosis)
- Use appropriate evidence-based assessment techniques and instruments in collecting data, including valid and reliable instruments that assess the high-incidence problem areas (e.g., distress thermometer).

Standard II. Diagnosis
- Use evidence-based research to formulate the plan of care.

Standard III. Outcome Identification
- Develop expected outcomes for each of the high-incidence problem areas at a level consistent with the patient's physical, psychological, social, and spiritual capacities, cultural background, and value system.
  - Comfort: Describe appropriate interventions for potential or predictable problems, such as pain, fatigue, dyspnea, sleep pattern disturbances, nausea, vomiting, and pruritus.
  - Mobility: The patient and/or family
    * Describe optimal levels of activities of daily living at a level consistent with disease state and treatment.
    * Identify health services and community resources available for managing changes in mobility.

Standard IV. Planning
- Develop the plan of care in collaboration with the patient, family, interdisciplinary cancer care team, and other healthcare professionals when possible.

Standard V. Implementation
- Use evidence-based research to guide implementation of interventions.

Standard VI. Evaluation
- Communicate the patient's response with the interdisciplinary cancer care team and other agencies involved in the healthcare continuum.

Figure 11-1. Standards Applicable to Physical Activity for Promoting Sleep

Note. From *Statement on the Scope and Standards of Oncology Nursing Practice: Generalist and Advanced Practice,* by J.M. Brant and R. Wickham (Eds.), 2013, Pittsburgh, PA: Oncology Nursing Society. Copyright 2013 by Oncology Nursing Society. Adapted with permission.

Sleep and Cancer-Related Sleep Disturbances

Sleep is defined as a reversible state in which individuals are behaviorally disengaged and unresponsive to their environment (Carskadon & Dement, 2011). Adults normally sleep seven to nine hours (420–540 minutes) in a 24-hour period. The human body performs best when it is active during the wake period and obtains deep sleep. The 24-hour sleep-wake cycle influences the regulation of the immune-inflammatory response (Besedovsky, Lange, & Born, 2012). The sleep-wake cycle also affects interactions among the central nervous, endocrine, and immune systems (Reis et al., 2011). Key parameters of sleep and their definitions are outlined in Table 11-1. The most basic information about sleep includes sleep latency, minutes awake after initial sleep onset, total sleep time, and sleep efficiency.

Table 11-1. Sleep Parameters Recommended for Evaluation of Sleep-Wake Disturbances

Parameter	Definition	Normal Range for Adults
Sleep quality	Subjective assessment of quality of sleep (very good to very poor)	Very good to very poor
Total sleep time	Number of hours or minutes of sleep in bed	7–9 hours (420–540 minutes)
Sleep latency	Number of minutes between getting into bed and falling asleep	Less than 30 minutes
Awakenings	Number of awakenings during the sleep period	2–6 brief awakenings
Wake after sleep onset	Number of minutes awake after initial sleep onset	Less than 30 minutes or less than 10% of sleep period
Daytime napping	Number of minutes of sleep during daytime naps	Less than 60 minutes
Daytime sleepiness	Number of episodes of falling asleep without intention	–
Circadian activity rhythms	Biobehavioral phenomenon that repeats approximately every 24 hours	Varies according to specific rhythm
Sleep efficiency	Number of minutes of sleep divided by the number of minutes in bed	85% or less

Note. Based on information from Berger et al., 2005.

Insomnia is defined as repeated difficulty with sleep initiation, duration, consolidation, or quality that occurs despite adequate time and opportunity for sleep, resulting in some form of daytime impairment. The three components of insomnia are inadequate sleep opportunity, persistent sleep difficulty, and associated daytime dysfunction (American Academy of Sleep Medicine, 2014).

Insomnia is the most common sleep disorder in the general public. Insomnia symptoms arise from primary causes and from medical illnesses such as cancer, mental health conditions, and other sleep disorders. Evidence suggests that even when insomnia appears secondary to another condition, it develops an independent course and often continues to be a clinically significant problem, even when the primary illness is treated adequately. Successful treatment of insomnia may improve both the sleep disturbance and other illnesses (American Academy of Sleep Medicine, 2014). Insomnia and other common adult sleep disorders are described in Table 11-2. Undiagnosed sleep disorders need to be identified by routine screening, and referral for sleep treatment should occur early in the cancer trajectory.

Effects of Cancer and Treatment on Sleep

Cancer and cancer treatments may disrupt the body's sleep-wake cycle, alter the body's immune-inflammatory responses, and modify interactions among sleep systems. Disruptions precipitate sleep-wake disturbances, particularly in adults who are predisposed to sleep disturbances, and can lead to attitudes and behaviors that perpetuate chronic insomnia (Spielman & Glovinsky, 2004).

During cancer treatment, sleep disturbances may occur from the following:
• Surgery and during the postoperative period
• Pain and immobility
• During chemotherapy due to forced hydration, symptoms, side effects, and adjuvant medications
• During and after radiation therapy

Impaired sleep quality, latency, total sleep time, and awakenings may predate chemotherapy treatment, worsen over the course of treatment, and persist after chemotherapy ends (Ancoli-Israel et al., 2014; Savard et al., 2009; Savard, Ivers, Savard, & Morin, 2015; Van Onselen et al., 2013). Therefore, sleep patterns and behaviors need to be assessed before, during, and after cancer treatment.

Benefits of Physical Activity and Exercise With Sleep

According to the U.S. Department of Health and Human Services (2008), evidence from a small number of studies demonstrates that regular partici-

Table 11-2. Common Sleep Disorders in Adults

Sleep Disorder	Definition	Presenting Symptoms	Recommendation
Insomnia	Difficulty initiating or maintaining sleep; causes significant impairment or distress for one month or more	Patient complains of difficulty falling asleep or staying asleep, or early morning awakening that impairs daytime function.	• Screening, assessment, diagnosis, and treatment • Set a regular bedtime and wake time. • Avoid napping within 1–4 hours before bedtime. • Avoid strenuous exercise immediately before main sleep period if this results in prolonged sleep latency or restless sleep.
Obstructive sleep apnea	Recurrent episodes of partial or complete upper airway obstruction (lasting 10–60 seconds) despite ongoing respiratory effort during sleep	Bed partner notices that patient stops breathing while asleep; often associated with snoring and excessive daytime sleepiness and non-refreshing sleep.	• Screening, assessment, diagnosis, and treatment • Adhere to prescribed obstructive sleep apnea treatment to obtain restful sleep and wake up refreshed. • Maintain a routine schedule for exercise and physical activity. • Maintain healthy body weight; lose weight if indicated.
Narcolepsy	Uncontrollable sleepiness and intermittent signs of rapid eye movement sleep that interrupt normal wakefulness	Patient reports suddenly falling asleep during usual activities.	• Screening, assessment, diagnosis, and treatment • Adhere to prescribed treatment to avoid injury while exercising.
Restless legs syndrome	Unpleasant urge or sensations in legs at night relieved by movement of limbs	Patient describes feelings of creeping, tingling, or cramping pain in legs that worsens when patient is lying down or at rest, particularly at the end of the day.	• Screening, assessment, diagnosis, and treatment • Adhere to prescribed treatment. • Maintain a routine schedule for exercise and physical activity. • Establish normal hemoglobin, hematocrit, and serum iron levels.

(Continued on next page)

Table 11-2. Common Sleep Disorders in Adults *(Continued)*

Sleep Disorder	Definition	Presenting Symptoms	Recommendation
Periodic limb movement disorder	Periodic or random kicking or arm movements during sleep	Bed partner reports kicking or arm movements by patient during sleep.	• Screening, assessment, diagnosis, and treatment • Adhere to prescribed treatment. • Maintain a schedule for exercise and physical activity. • Set a regular bedtime and wake time.
Circadian rhythm disorder	Major sleep episode is advanced or delayed in relation to desired clock time and results in undesired insomnia or sleepiness	Patient reports inability to fall asleep or awaken relative to conventional sleep-wake times.	• Screening, assessment, diagnosis, and treatment • Maintain regular sleep patterns. • Maintain a schedule for exercise and physical activity.
Parasomnia	Undesirable physical events or behaviors that occur during entry into sleep, within sleep, or during arousals from sleep	Bed partner reports behaviors by patient such as sleepwalking, sleep talking, or sleep terrors.	• Screening, assessment, diagnosis, and treatment • Adhere to prescribed treatment. • Maintain a schedule for exercise/physical activity.
Hypersomnia	Constant or recurrent episodes of extreme sleepiness during the wake period	Patient reports daily periods of irrepressible need to sleep or daytime lapses into sleep occurring for at least three months.	• Screening, assessment, diagnosis, and treatment • Adhere to prescribed treatment. • Maintain a schedule for exercise and physical activity.

Note. Based on information from American Academy of Sleep Medicine, 2014; National Sleep Foundation, 2011.

pation in physical activity has favorable effects on sleep quality and is a useful component of good sleep hygiene. The National Sleep Foundation (2013) recommends regular exercise to improve sleep. Although vigorous exercise is best, even light exercise is better than no activity (National Sleep Foundation, 2013).

Empirical and anecdotal evidence suggests that healthy adults with sleep problems and those with cancer who engage in physical activity and exercise experi-

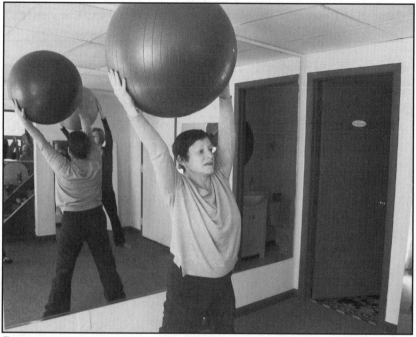

Exercise can improve sleep in cancer survivors.

ence improved sleep quality (Chiu, Huang, Chen, Hou, & Tsai, 2015; Yang, Ho, Chen, & Chien, 2012). A number of studies have examined the therapeutic value of physical activity and exercise on sleep during and after primary cancer treatment. Most studies investigated women with early-stage breast cancer receiving chemotherapy or radiation therapy, and several examined men and women with mixed types of diagnoses. Table 11-3 summarizes examples of research studies related to the effect of physical activity and exercise on sleep in cancer survivors.

Cardiovascular/Aerobic Exercise

Two recent reviews and meta-analyses synthesized the cumulative evidence regarding endurance/aerobic exercise in cancer survivors (Chiu et al., 2015; Langford, Lee, & Miaskowski, 2012). The most common intervention was home-based walking. Chiu et al.'s systematic review suggested that moderate-intensity walking exercise is likely to be effective in improving sleep in individuals with cancer. Langford et al.'s findings showed a positive trend but were inconclusive. Two other meta-analyses (Mishra, Scherer, Geigle, et al., 2012; Mishra, Scherer, Snyder, et al., 2012) reported that exercise improved sleep in adults with cancer during and after treatment; however, their conclusions have been questioned (Chiu et al., 2015).

Table 11-3. Research Exemplars for Physical Activity and Exercise to Promote Sleep in Cancer Survivors

Type	Description	Goal	Exemplar Studies in Cancer Survivors
Cardiovascular	Aerobic activity such as brisk walking, jogging, and cycling	Increase breathing, heart rate, and overall fitness	In a study by Tang et al. (2010), 71 Taiwanese adults (mean age = 58 years) with mixed cancers, predominantly breast cancer (n = 62), who complained of sleep problems attended 16 hours of classes over 6–8 weeks to learn home-based brisk walking tailored to their individual rate of perceived exertion. Their goal was 30 minutes of exercise 3 days per week. Sleep was measured by the Pittsburgh Sleep Quality Index (PSQI). Participants in the exercise group had significant improvement in sleep quality (p < 0.01) at 1 and 2 months compared to usual care.
Strengthening	Strength training such as water aerobics and weights; resistance training (e.g., resistance bands)	Improve muscle strength	In a study by Rajotte et al. (2012), 187 self-referred adults with mixed cancers who were at least 90 days post-treatment (predominantly female; mean age = 58 years) attended 90-minute sessions, twice per week over 12 weeks. The participants had supervised individual resistance training by personal trainers in a group setting at 13 YMCA sites. They participated in a 10-minute aerobic warm-up followed by resistance training. Sleep was measured by a 3-item Likert insomnia rating scale (0–4). Subjective rating of insomnia declined from baseline to 12 weeks (p < 0.001).

(Continued on next page)

Table 11-3. Research Exemplars for Physical Activity and Exercise to Promote Sleep in Cancer Survivors *(Continued)*

Type	Description	Goal	Exemplar Studies in Cancer Survivors
Balance	Balance training such as tai chi Qigong or lower-body strength training	Improve balance and prevent falls	In a study by Fong et al. (2015), 52 nasopharyngeal cancer survivors in Hong Kong (mean age = 58 years) who had completed chemotherapy or radiation therapy attended 6 months of tai chi Qigong training for 90-minute sessions, four times per week, including home practice. The Medical Outcomes Study Sleep Scale measured sleep problems. Compared to usual care, sleep problems decreased in the tai chi Qigong group ($p < 0.008$), and this effect was greatest at 6 months; improvement in cervical side flexion range of motion was associated with a reduction in sleep problems in the tai chi Qigong group ($p < 0.05$).
Flexibility	Flexibility training such as yoga	Stretch muscles and improve freedom of movement	In a study by Mustian et al. (2013), 410 cancer survivors (mean age = 54 years) with mixed cancer types (75% breast cancer) and moderate to severe insomnia participated in supervised exercise sessions. The survivors were 2–24 months posttreatment, and the group was predominantly (> 90%) female. The participants attended 75-minute sessions twice per week over 4 weeks. Yoga intervention consisted of breathing exercises, gentle Hatha yoga, restorative yoga postures, and meditation. Sleep was measured by the PSQI, actigraphy (24 hours/7 days), and sleep medication use pre- and postintervention. Compared to usual care, the yoga group showed greater improvements in sleep quality, daytime dysfunction, wake after sleep onset, sleep efficiency, and reduction in medication use at postintervention ($p < 0.05$).

Randomized controlled trials (RCTs) testing tailored endurance and aerobic exercise in adults have reported mixed results. The exemplar study in Table 11-3 tested endurance exercise and found significant improvement in sleep quality compared to usual care (p < 0.01) (Tang, Liou, & Lin, 2010). Higher volumes of aerobic exercise were found to be superior to a standard dose for managing global sleep quality in patients with breast cancer receiving chemotherapy (Courneya et al., 2014). In contrast, studies in lymphoma (Courneya et al., 2012), breast, colorectal, or ovarian cancer (Dodd et al., 2010), and mixed solid tumors (Wenzel et al., 2013) did not report significantly improved sleep quality as assessed by the Pittsburgh Sleep Quality Index (PSQI) or General Sleep Disturbance Scale.

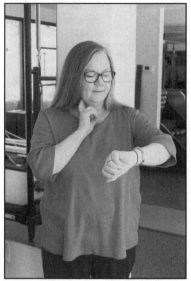

Cancer survivors can determine the desired intensity of their workout by checking their pulse during exercise.

Strength/Resistance Exercise

Studies of resistance or strength training have included use of resistance bands combined with an endurance/aerobic component. The exemplar study conducted in a community-based exercise program at 13 YMCAs reported that subjective insomnia ratings declined from baseline to postintervention (p < 0.001) (Rajotte, Baker, Gregerson, Leiserowitz, & Syrjala, 2012). This finding suggests that community exercise groups for cancer survivors of mixed diagnoses and ages can improve sleep and are safe. Results of other studies that included resistance are mixed. In patients with advanced lung and colorectal cancer who received a 90-minute walking and resistance-band training session and bimonthly phone follow-ups, sleep ratings (on a 0–10 numeric rating scale) improved compared to usual care (Cheville et al., 2013). The effect of a 12-week, home-based resistance band and walking intervention on sleep measured by actigraphy was examined in 187 patients with newly diagnosed multiple myeloma during active chemotherapy and transplant treatment (Coleman et al., 2012). Over the course of treatment, participants' status declined, and they experienced greater fatigue, shorter total sleep time, and shorter distances on a six-minute walk test. No differences were reported in night or daytime sleep time or efficiency between the intervention and usual care groups, possibly due to the inconsistent intensity of the intervention because of different cancer treatments.

Flexibility Exercise

Studies investigating the efficacy of a flexibility-type exercise on sleep during and after cancer treatment have focused primarily on yoga and on women with breast cancer. A systematic review of 13 studies examining the effects of various yoga modalities found that only one study included a sleep outcome, which was not improved with yoga intervention (Sharma, Haider, & Knowlden, 2013). Similarly, a meta-analysis of six RCTs reported no significant effect of yoga on sleep improvement (Zhang, Yang, Tian, & Wang, 2012). Alexander and Lockwood (2014) conducted a systematic review on the effectiveness of a yoga practice on sleep quality in adult patients with cancer. Of the five randomized clinical trials reviewed, three found that patients who practiced yoga had less sleep disturbances and insomnia compared to those who did not practice yoga. The exemplar of a flexibility exercise study by Mustian et al. (2013) is the largest RCT (N = 413) that tested yoga. The intervention consisted of breathing exercises, gentle Hatha yoga, and restorative yoga postures and meditation (Mustian et al., 2013). Those who attended group yoga sessions self-reported improved global sleep quality (via the PSQI) and less daytime dysfunction postintervention, but results from actigraphy data did not demonstrate differences between groups.

Balance

Only one study examined the effects of exercise to improve balance (tai chi Qigong) on sleep quality (Fong et al., 2015). Using the Medical Outcomes Study Sleep Scale, Fong et al. (2015) saw a decrease in sleep problems for patients with nasopharyngeal cancer who received tai chi Qigong training, suggesting that this intervention is effective in reducing sleep problems among nasopharyngeal cancer survivors.

Oncology Nursing Assessment

Self-Report and Sleep Screening Measures

1. Assess sleep quality using self-report and sleep screening measures. Assessing the cancer survivor's sleep quality is one component of an overall health assessment conducted by oncology nurses. Several well-established methods exist to self-rate sleep quality (see Table 11-4). Positive screening results indicate sleep disturbances, and additional assessment by the oncology team is warranted. A clinical review of systems, an in-depth interview, and additional screenings are indicated for appropriate diagnosis and treatment. Additional screening tools may include the STOP-Bang (Chung et al., 2008, 2012) for obstructive sleep apnea and the Epworth Sleepiness Scale (Johns, 1991) for excessive daytime sleepiness.

Table 11-4. Common Clinical Sleep-Wake Assessment Tools

Scale	Description	Other Information
Daily sleep diary	10–12 items (e.g., bedtime, awakenings, sleep quality ratings) self-reported for a minimum of one week to identify usual sleep patterns in a natural sleep environment	Individual to complete items each morning and discuss weekly entries with the oncology nurse to help detect sleep-wake patterns and circadian disturbances
Epworth Sleepiness Scale	8-item scale evaluating daytime sleepiness	Individual self-ratings of tendency to doze off in common situations (e.g., watching television, driving)
Pittsburgh Sleep Quality Index	19-item scale with 5 bed partner items to assess whether the patient's sleep is normal or aligns with several sleep disorders	Well-established tool that uses self-report to screen for insomnia and other sleep disorders; however, scoring cumbersome for clinical settings
Insomnia Severity Index	7-item brief and easy clinical method to screen for the severity and impact of insomnia	Individuals self-rate insomnia symptoms and consequences for two weeks; easily administered and scored
Clinical Sleep Assessment for Adults	Brief set of 7 sleep screening items useful for a clinic appointment	Clinical self-rating tool to assess sleep history, habits, bedtime routine, and nocturnal behaviors; easily administered and scored
Patient-Reported Outcomes Measurement System	Scales developed and validated by the National Institutes of Health with subscale items developed from a large, validated item bank	Reliable, precise measures of self-reported sleep disturbance and sleep-related impairment

Note. Based on information from Buysse et al., 1989; Carney et al., 2012; Gershon et al., 2010; Johns, 1991; Lee & Ward, 2005; Savard et al., 2005.

2. Obtain your oncology center's current sleep assessment scales. Review the questions you ask cancer survivors about their sleep patterns. Compare your center's practice with the assessments listed in this chapter.
3. Determine if a referral for sleep-related services is needed based on the self-assessment and screening.

Self-Report and Physical Activity/Exercise Assessment

1. Assess current physical activity and exercise patterns using measures such as those described in Chapter 4. Use the physical activity and exercise mea-

sures endorsed by your oncology center to measure activity. Assessing the cancer survivor's current physical activity and exercise program will help you understand the level of physical activity in which the survivor is currently engaged.

2. Evaluate the relationship between the cancer survivor's physical activity and exercise and sleep patterns. Use the FITT principle to assess the frequency, intensity, time, and type of activities. Are the activities performed later in the day related to the survivor's sleep patterns? Are the frequency and intensity of activities similar to the evidence presented in this chapter?

3. Review screenings as needed to determine physical readiness for exercise (see Chapter 7).

4. Determine if a consultation to a physical or occupational therapist is indicated to develop an individualized physical activity and exercise plan (NCCN, 2016).
   • Bed rest: Physical therapy exercises to maintain strength and range of motion to help counteract sleep disturbances, fatigue, and mood alterations are recommended.
   • Special health conditions: Survivors with bone disease, arthritis, or peripheral neuropathy require careful attention to balance and safety to reduce fall risk (see Chapters 12 and 13).

Oncology Nursing Recommendations for Physical Activity and Exercise to Promote Sleep

1. Use any of the interviewing techniques discussed in Chapter 5 to determine survivors' readiness to incorporate physical activity and exercise into their lifestyle.

2. Teach survivors about the potential benefits of physical activity and exercise on improving sleep. Use the evidence presented in this chapter to create an education fact sheet or revise the materials provided by your oncology center. Assure survivors that an individualized physical activity and exercise plan has been shown to be safe for promoting sleep during and after cancer treatment.

3. Use interventions to reduce cancer-related symptom severity and distress, including sleep disturbances (Berger, Desaulniers, Matthews, Otte, & Page, 2014; Berger et al., 2015).

4. Collaborate with cancer survivors to select physical activities and exercises they enjoy and are able to perform regularly and safely. Use checklists offered by your oncology center.

5. Use the FITT principle to collaborate with survivors and create a physical activity and exercise plan. Incorporating a variety of exercise types reduces boredom and risk of repetitive injury (National Institute on Aging, 2015).

6. Consider chemotherapy treatment schedules, blood counts, surgery-related restrictions, and other health-related factors when creating a physical activity plan.
7. Calculate the target heart rate zone. Teach survivors how to measure their heart rate and rating of perceived exertion.
8. Provide a discharge packet for physical activity and exercise to promote sleep that includes the following (see Chapter 8):
   • Sleep diary to record sleep quantity and quality
   • Insomnia Severity Index to rate sleep and daytime functioning
9. Set short-term (daily or weekly) and long-term (monthly) goals with cancer survivors and their families for physical activity and exercise to gradually reach 150 minutes of aerobic activity per week (Jankowski & Matthews, 2011).
10. Encourage survivors to report moderate to severe symptoms after starting physical activity and exercise to discuss ways to reduce these symptoms.
11. Select a method for tracking physical activity and sleep patterns. Ask survivors to bring the tracking program with them on their next visit.
12. Recommend support systems, such as a walking partner or group, and resources, including indoor walking facilities, to initiate and maintain an active physical activity and exercise plan.

Oncology Nursing Evaluation of Health Outcomes

1. Evaluate cancer survivors' adherence to the recommended physical activity/exercise plan by discussing their self-report outcomes.
2. Evaluate these outcomes to the plan adherence and their sleep patterns. Note any improvements in or worsening of sleep patterns.
3. Discuss with survivors their experiences with the physical activity and exercise plan and their sleep patterns. Use the interviewing techniques in Chapter 5.
4. Revise the physical activity and exercise plan as needed according to the effects of the plan on cancer-related symptoms. Adjust the frequency, intensity, time, and type of activities to meet survivors' needs for sleep and other symptom management.
5. Follow up with referrals for sleep evaluation, physical or occupational therapy, and exercise testing as required by your oncology center.

Application to Oncology Nursing Practice

1. Sleep pattern assessment is an important component of oncology nursing.

2. Synthesizing sleep assessments with psychosocial and physical readiness for physical activity and exercise allows oncology nurses to determine a safe approach for creating feasible activity plans.
3. Oncology nurses and their patients can use the FITT principle to create an achievable physical activity plan.
4. Evaluating health outcomes at subsequent visits allows oncology nurses to analyze the effects of physical activity plans on sleep and other health-related outcomes during and after cancer treatment.

Summary

Despite methodologic limitations, meta-analyses, reviews, and individual studies support the general benefits of exercise in improving sleep in cancer survivors. Recent evidence suggests that exercise is likely to be effective in improving sleep, is acceptable and feasible, and can maintain or improve physical functioning in patients. Larger, well-designed RCTs are needed to determine the long-term effectiveness of different types of exercise on sleep in a variety of cancer populations, and to delineate predictors of exercise effectiveness (e.g., frequency, intensity, timing, adherence rates) on outcomes.

Oncology nurses can use existing resources to strengthen their confidence in recommending physical activity for promoting sleep and managing cancer-related symptoms:
• NCCN Guidelines®: www.nccn.org
• Oncology Nursing Society's Putting Evidence Into Practice resources: www.ons.org/practice-resources/pep
• Berger, A.M., Desaulniers, G., Matthews, E.E., Otte, J.L., & Page, M.S. (2014). Sleep-wake disturbances. In M. Irwin & L.A. Johnson (Eds.), *Putting evidence into practice: A pocket guide to cancer symptom management* (pp. 255–267). Pittsburgh, PA: Oncology Nursing Society.

Oncology nurses are well-positioned to promote healthy sleep using safe and effective physical activities and exercises supported by the literature as well as survivor preferences.

Case Study

G.G. is a 65-year-old woman who was diagnosed with stage IIIC colorectal cancer (T3 N2 M0). After a right hemicolectomy, she received the FOLFOX chemotherapy regimen (oxaliplatin, leucovorin, and 5-fluorouracil) for six months. When she completed her FOLFOX treatment, she complained of insomnia, fatigue, and daytime dysfunction. G.G. works as a receptionist at a hair salon and took time off during treatment. Last month, she worked two to three days per week at the end of treatment. She is divorced with two grown children and lives alone. She often babysits her three granddaughters. She has never smoked and rarely drinks alcohol. She was physically active in her twenties and thirties but has been sedentary since then due to work and family responsibilities. Before her cancer diagnosis and treatment, her activities included shopping, doing household chores, and light gardening. G.G. does not feel safe walking alone in her neighborhood. G.G. reports problems with physical and mental functioning throughout the day. She has trouble falling asleep and staying asleep at night (see Figure 11-2).

Height/weight	• Height: 5'2" • Weight: 160 lbs • BMI: 29.3 • Overweight
Vitals	• Blood pressure: 150/84 mm Hg • Resting heart rate: 88 bpm • Respiratory rate: 22 breaths per minute • Temperature: 98.6°F (37°C)
Cardiopulmonary	• Normal lung sounds bilaterally • Normal cardiovascular examination
Other	• Karnofsky Performance Scale status: 90% (able to carry on regular activity; minor symptoms of disease) • Bowel sounds present and normal in all quadrants

Figure 11-2. Additional Patient Information

BMI—body mass index; bpm—beats per minute

Relevant Laboratory Values
• Hemoglobin: 10 g/dl
• Hematocrit: 30%

Medical History
• Hypertension
• Arthritis

Medications
• Lisinopril
• Acetaminophen PRN for joint pain

Insomnia Management Plan

• Establish a regular bedtime and wake time (7–9 hours/night).
• Avoid daytime napping if it affects sleep onset or maintenance.
• Manage other symptoms (e.g., anemia, arthritis pain).
• Establish a pattern of exercise in divided sessions but not too close to bedtime, as it may interfere with sleep onset.
• Avoid stimulants (e.g., coffee, cola) in the evening.

Physical Activity Management Plan

- Encourage patient to enroll in an exercise program for cancer survivors at local YWCA with personal trainer.
- Determine target training heart rate (HR) using Karvonen formula:
  1. Maximum HR (MHR) = 220 (constant) − 65 (patient's age) = 155 beats per minute (bpm)
  2. HR reserve = 155 (MHR) − 88 (resting HR [RHR]) = 67 bpm
  3. Initial desired exercise intensity = light to moderate (40% of training heart rate)
  4. Target training HR = 67 (HR reserve) × 0.40 (desired intensity) + 88 (RHR) = 115 bpm

---

Sample Initial Exercise Prescription

Exercise Type	Frequency	Intensity	Time	Type
Strength training	2 times per week	One set, 8–10 reps to start, with light weights	8–10 exercises addressing major muscle groups	Begin with body weight exercises and progress to free weights (i.e., dumbbells) or machine weights.
Cardiovascular	3 times per week	Light to start (up to 50% maximum heart rate or rating of perceived exertion of 2–3/10) Individual should be able to easily talk during exercise without feeling out of breath (see Table 4-3 in Chapter 4).	20–30 minutes of sustained exercise	Walking
Flexibility	During warm-up and cooldown	To the point of light resistance	5–10 minutes	Stretching large muscle groups

Follow-Up

After six months, G.G.'s rating of perceived exertion during endurance exercise has decreased from 15 (hard) to 11 (light). She usually reaches a target training heart rate of 100–110 bpm and is gradually working toward 115 bpm. G.G.'s total minutes of aerobic activity per week has increased from 0 to 75 minutes, and she now does strength training with weights twice per week and flexibility and balance training five times per week.

G.G. self-reports the following after one week:
- Decrease in minutes awake after sleep onset (from 100 to 45)
- Improved sleep efficiency (from 75% to 85%)
- Decreased Insomnia Severity Index score (from 18 to 14)
- Decreased self-reported sleep problem interference with daily functioning (e.g., daytime fatigue, ability to function at work or during daily chores, concentration, memory, mood)

References

Alexander, G.K., & Lockwood, S. (2014). Effect of yoga on sleep quality among adult cancer patients: A systematic review. *JBI Database of Systematic Reviews and Implementation Reports, 12,* 382–419. doi:10.11124/jbisrir-2014-1654

American Academy of Sleep Medicine. (2014). *International classification of sleep disorders* (3rd ed.). Darien, IL: American Academy of Sleep Medicine.

American Council on Exercise. (2003). *ACE personal trainer manual* (3rd ed.). San Diego, CA: Author.

Ancoli-Israel, S., Liu, L., Rissling, M., Natarajan, L., Neikrug, A.B., Palmer, B.W., & Maglione, J. (2014). Sleep, fatigue, depression, and circadian activity rhythms in women with breast cancer before and after treatment: A 1-year longitudinal study. *Supportive Care in Cancer, 22,* 2535–2545. doi:10.1007/s00520-014-2204-5

Berger, A.M., Desaulniers, G., Matthews, E.E., Otte, J.L., & Page, M.S. (2014). Sleep-wake disturbances. In M. Irwin & L.A. Johnson (Eds.), *Putting evidence into practice: A pocket guide to cancer symptom management* (pp. 255–267). Pittsburgh, PA: Oncology Nursing Society.

Berger, A.M., Desaulniers, G., Matthews, E.E., Otte, J.L., Page, M.S., & Vena, C. (2015). Putting evidence into practice: Sleep-wake disturbances. Retrieved from https://www.ons.org/practice-resources/pep/sleep-wake-disturbances

Berger, A.M., Parker, K.P., Young-McCaughan, S., Mallory, G.A., Barsevick, A.M., Beck, S.L., ... Hall, M. (2005). Sleep/wake disturbances in people with cancer and their caregivers: State of the science [Online exclusive]. *Oncology Nursing Forum, 32,* E98–E126. doi:10.1188/05.ONF.E98-E126

Besedovsky, L., Lange, T., & Born, J. (2012). Sleep and immune function. *Pflügers Archiv, 463,* 121–137. doi:10.1007/s00424-011-1044-0

Brant, J.M., & Wickham, R. (Eds.). (2013). *Statement on the scope and standards of oncology nursing practice: Generalist and advanced practice.* Pittsburgh, PA: Oncology Nursing Society.

Buysse, D., Reynolds, C.F., Monk, T.H., Berman, S.R., & Kupfer, D.J. (1989). The Pittsburgh Sleep Quality Index: A new instrument for psychiatric practice and research. *Psychiatry Research, 28,* 193–213. doi:10.1016/0165-1781(89)90047-4

Carney, C.E., Buysse, D.J., Ancoli-Israel, S., Edinger, J.D., Krystal, A.D., Lichstein, K.L., & Morin, C.M. (2012). The Consensus Sleep Diary: Standardizing prospective sleep self-monitoring. *Sleep, 35,* 287–302. doi:10.5665/sleep.1642

Carskadon, M., & Dement, W.C. (2011). Normal human sleep: An overview. In M.H. Kryer, T. Roth, & W.C. Dement (Eds.), *Principles and practice of sleep medicine* (5th ed., pp. 16–26). Philadelphia, PA: Elsevier Saunders.

Cheville, A.L., Kollasch, J., Vandenberg, J., Shen, T., Grothey, A., Gamble, G., & Basford, J.R. (2013). A home-based exercise program to improve function, fatigue, and sleep quality in patients with stage IV lung and colorectal cancer: A randomized controlled trial. *Journal of Pain and Symptom Management, 45,* 811–821. doi:10.1016/j.jpainsymman.2012.05.006

Chiu, H.-Y., Huang, H.-C., Chen, P.-Y., Hou, W.-H., & Tsai, P.-S. (2015). Walking improves sleep in individuals with cancer: A meta-analysis of randomized, controlled trials [Online exclusive]. *Oncology Nursing Forum, 42,* E54–E62. doi:10.1188/15.ONF.E54-E62

Chung, F., Subramanyam, R., Liao, P., Sasaki, E., Shapiro, C., & Sun, Y. (2012). High STOP-Bang score indicates a high probability of obstructive sleep apnea. *British Journal of Anaesthesia, 108,* 768–775. doi:10.1093/bja/aes022

Chung, F., Yegneswaran, B., Liao, P., Chung, S.A., Vairavanathan, S., Islam, S., ... Shapiro, C.M. (2008). STOP questionnaire: A tool to screen patients for obstructive sleep apnea. *Anesthesiology, 108,* 812–821. doi:10.1097/ALN.0b013e31816d83e4

Coleman, E.A., Goodwin, J.A., Kennedy, R., Coon, S.K., Richards, K., Enderlin, C., ... Anaissie, E.J. (2012). Effects of exercise on fatigue, sleep, and performance: A randomized trial. *Oncology Nursing Forum, 39,* 468–477. doi:10.1188/12.ONF.468-477

Courneya, K.S., Segal, R.J., Mackey, J.R., Gelmon, K., Friedenreich, C.M., Yasui, Y., ... McKenzie, D.C. (2014). Effects of exercise dose and type on sleep quality in breast cancer patients receiving chemotherapy: A multicenter randomized trial. *Breast Cancer Research and Treatment, 144,* 361–369. doi:10.1007/s10549-014-2883-0

Courneya, K.S., Sellar, C.M., Trinh, L., Forbes, C.C., Stevinson, C., McNeely, M.L., ... Reiman, T. (2012). A randomized trial of aerobic exercise and sleep quality in lymphoma patients receiving chemotherapy or no treatment. *Cancer Epidemiology, Biomarkers and Prevention, 21,* 887–894. doi:10.1158/1055-9965.EPI-12-0075

Dodd, M.J., Cho, M.H., Miaskowski, C., Painter, P.L., Paul, S.M., Cooper, B.A., ... Bank, K.A. (2010). A randomized controlled trial of home-based exercise for cancer-related fatigue in women during and after chemotherapy with or without radiation therapy. *Cancer Nursing, 33,* 245–257. doi:10.1097/NCC.0b013e3181ddc58c

Fong, S.S.M., Ng, S.S.M., Lee, H.W., Pang, M.Y.C., Luk, W.S., Chung, J.W.Y., ... Masters, R.S.W. (2015). The effects of a 6-month Tai Chi Qigong training program on temporomandibular, cervical, and shoulder joint mobility and sleep problems in nasopharyngeal cancer survivors. *Integrative Cancer Therapies, 14,* 16–25. doi:10.1177/1534735414556508

Gershon, R.C., Rothrock, N., Hanrahan, R., Bass, M., & Cella, D. (2010). The use of PROMIS and assessment center to deliver patient-reported outcome measures in clinical research. *Journal of Applied Measurement, 11,* 304–314.

Jankowski, C.M., & Matthews, E.E. (2011). Exercise guidelines for adults with cancer: A vital role in survivorship. *Clinical Journal of Oncology Nursing, 15,* 683–686. doi:10.1188/11.CJON.683-686

Johns, M.W. (1991). A new method for measuring daytime sleepiness: The Epworth Sleepiness Scale. *Sleep, 14,* 540–545. Retrieved from http://epworthsleepinessscale.com/wp-content/uploads/2008/12/a-new-method-for-measuring-daytime-sleepiness-the-epworth-sleepiness-scale2.pdf

Langford, D.J., Lee, K., & Miaskowski, C. (2012). Sleep disturbance interventions in oncology patients and family caregivers: A comprehensive review and meta-analysis. *Sleep Medicine Reviews, 16,* 397–414. doi:10.1016/j.smrv.2011.07.002

Lee, K.A., & Ward, T.M. (2005). Critical components of a sleep assessment for clinical practice settings. *Issues in Mental Health Nursing, 26,* 739–750. doi:10.1080/01612840591008320

Mishra, S.I., Scherer, R.W., Geigle, P.M., Berlanstein, D.R., Topaloglu, O., Gotay, C.C., & Snyder, C. (2012). Exercise interventions on health-related quality of life for cancer survivors. *Cochrane Database of Systematic Reviews, 2012*(8). doi:10.1002/14651858.CD007566.pub2

Mishra, S.I., Scherer, R.W., Snyder, C., Geigle, P.M., Berlanstein, D.R., & Topaloglu, O. (2012). Exercise interventions on health-related quality of life for people with cancer during active treatment. *Cochrane Database of Systematic Reviews, 2012*(8). doi:10.1002/14651858.CD008465. pub2

Mustian, K.M., Sprod, L.K., Janelsins, M., Peppone, L.J., Palesh, O.G., Chandwani, K., ... Morrow, G.R. (2013). Multicenter, randomized controlled trial of yoga for sleep quality among cancer survivors. *Journal of Clinical Oncology, 31*, 3233–3241. doi:10.1200/JCO.2012.43.7707

National Comprehensive Cancer Network. (2015). *NCCN Clinical Practice Guidelines in Oncology (NCCN Guidelines®): Survivorship* [v.2.2015]. Retrieved from http://www.nccn.org/professionals/physician_gls/pdf/pain.pdf

National Comprehensive Cancer Network. (2016). *NCCN Clinical Practice Guidelines in Oncology (NCCN Guidelines®): Cancer-related pain* [v.1.2016]. Retrieved from http://www.nccn.org/professionals/physician_gls/pdf/fatigue.pdf

National Institute on Aging. (2015). Go4Life. Retrieved from https://go4life.nia.nih.gov

National Sleep Foundation. (2011). Insomnia. Retrieved from http://www.sleepfoundation.org/article/sleep-related-problems/insomnia-and-sleep

National Sleep Foundation. (2013). National Sleep Foundation poll finds exercise key to good sleep. Retrieved from https://sleepfoundation.org/media-center/national-sleep-foundation-poll-finds-exercise-key/page/0/2

Rajotte, E.J., Yi, J.C., Baker, K.S., Gregerson, L., Leiserowitz, A., & Syrjala, K.L. (2012). Community-based exercise program effectiveness and safety for cancer survivors. *Journal of Cancer Survivorship, 6*, 219–228. doi:10.1007/s11764-011-0213-7

Reis, E.S., Lange, T., Köhl, G., Herrmann, A., Tschulakow, A.V., Naujoks, J., ... Köhl, J. (2011). Sleep and circadian rhythm regulate circulating complement factors and immunoregulatory properties of C5a. *Brain, Behavior, and Immunity, 25*, 1416–1426. doi:10.1016/j.bbi.2011.04.011

Savard, J., Ivers, H., Savard, M.H., & Morin, C.M. (2015). Cancer treatments and their side effects are associated with aggravation of insomnia: Results of a longitudinal study. *Cancer, 121*, 1703–1711. doi:10.1002/cncr.29244

Savard, J., Liu, L., Natarajan, L., Rissling, M.B., Neikrug, A.B., He, F., ... Ancoli-Israel, S. (2009). Breast cancer patients have progressively impaired sleep-wake activity rhythms during chemotherapy. *Sleep, 32*, 1155–1160.

Savard, M., Savard, J., Simard, S., & Ivers, H. (2005). Empirical validation of the Insomnia Severity Index in cancer patients. *Psycho-Oncology, 14*, 429–441. doi:10.1002/pon.860

Schmitz, K.H., Courneya, K.S., Matthews, C., Demark-Wahnefried, W., Galvão, D.A., Pinto, B.M., ... Schwartz, A.L. (2010). American College of Sports Medicine roundtable on exercise guidelines for cancer survivors. *Medicine and Science in Sports and Exercise, 42*, 1409–1426. doi:10.1249/MSS.0b013e3181e0c112

Sharma, M., Haider, T., & Knowlden, A.P. (2013). Yoga as an alternative and complementary treatment for cancer: A systematic review. *Journal of Alternative and Complementary Medicine, 19*, 870–875. doi:10.1089/acm.2012.0632

Spielman, A.J., & Glovinsky, P.B. (2004). A conceptual framework of insomnia for primary care practitioners: Predisposing, precipitating and perpetuating factors. *Sleep Medicine Alerts, 9*, 1–6.

Tang, M.-F., Liou, T.-H., & Lin, C.-C. (2010). Improving sleep quality for cancer patients: Benefits of a home-based exercise intervention. *Supportive Care in Cancer, 18*, 1329–1339. doi:10.1007/s00520-009-0757-5

U.S. Department of Health and Human Services. (2008). *Physical Activity Guidelines Advisory Committee report. Part G. Section 8: Mental health.* Retrieved from http://health.gov/paguidelines/report/g8_mentalhealth.aspx#_Toc197778637

Van Onselen, C., Paul, S.M., Lee, K., Dunn, L., Aouizerat, B.E., West, C., ... Miaskowski, C. (2013). Trajectories of sleep disturbance and daytime sleepiness in women before and after surgery for breast cancer. *Journal of Pain and Symptom Management, 45*, 244–260. doi:10.1016/j.jpainsymman.2012.02.020

Wenzel, J.A., Griffith, K.A., Shang, J., Thompson, C.B., Hedlin, H., Stewart, K.J., ... Mock, V. (2013). Impact of a home-based walking intervention on outcomes of sleep quality, emotional distress, and fatigue in patients undergoing treatment for solid tumors. *Oncologist, 18*, 476–484. doi:10.1634/theoncologist.2012-0278

Yang, P.-Y., Ho, K.-H., Chen, H.-C., & Chien, M.-Y. (2012). Exercise training improves sleep quality in middle-aged and older adults with sleep problems: A systematic review. *Journal of Physiotherapy, 58*, 157–163. doi:10.1016/S1836-9553(12)70106-6

Zhang, J., Yang, K.-H., Tian, J.-H., & Wang, C.-M. (2012). Effects of yoga on psychologic function and quality of life in women with breast cancer: A meta-analysis of randomized controlled trials. *Journal of Alternative and Complementary Medicine, 18*, 994–1002. doi:10.1089/acm.2011.0514

CHAPTER 12

Physical Activity for Chronic Cancer-Related Conditions

Amy J. Litterini, PT, DPT

Introduction

Cancer survivors present with unique issues directly related to their cancer and treatment. Lymphedema, cachexia, and bone loss or fracture risk challenge oncology nurses to recommend safe and doable physical activities for cancer survivors experiencing these conditions. This chapter discusses common chronic cancer-related special considerations and offers guidance to create meaningful physical activity and exercise programs. Referral to trained oncology rehabilitation professionals is recommended for these special conditions. In addition, cancer-related emergencies are addressed. This chapter's content is supported in the Oncology Nursing Society's *Statement on the Scope and Standards of Oncology Nursing Practice: Generalist and Advanced Practice* (Brant & Wickham, 2013) (see Figure 12-1).

Lymphedema

In addition to its immune system function, the lymph system is considered an accessory route for the transportation of lymph fluid from the tissues into the bloodstream. In this role, the lymphatic system works with the cardiovascular system to maintain fluid balance throughout the body (Zuther & Norton, 2013). Disruption of this balance, caused by anatomic malformation or trauma, will result in lymphatic insufficiency, leading to local or generalized edema. Lymphatic insufficiency can be either *dynamic,* where both active and passive edema protective measures fail, or *mechanical,* where

---

Standard I. Assessment
- Collect data in the following high-incidence problem areas. These areas may include but are not limited to the following:
  - Mobility
    * Past and present level of mobility and overall function
    * Risk for decreased mobility
    * Impact of fatigue on mobility
    * Complications related to decreased mobility
  - Survivorship
    * Patient/family understanding of the potential late effects of cancer treatment (e.g., secondary malignancies, organ toxicities, altered fertility, osteoporosis) prior to initiation of therapy
    * Patient/family understanding of the potential persistent or long-term effects associated with cancer treatment (e.g., fatigue, taste changes, cognitive changes, osteoporosis)

Standard II. Diagnosis
- Use evidence-based research to formulate the plan of care.

Standard III. Outcome Identification
- Design expected outcomes to maximize the patient's functional abilities.
- Develop expected outcomes for each of the 14 high-incidence problem areas at a level consistent with the patient's physical, psychological, social, and spiritual capacities, cultural background, and value system. The expected outcomes include but are not limited to the following:
  - Mobility
    * Incorporate safety and fall prevention strategies in the mobility plan.
    * Explain the impact of fatigue on immobility.
    * Explain the relationship between fatigue and exercise balance.
    * Describe an appropriate management plan to integrate alteration in mobility into lifestyle.
    * Describe optimal levels of activities of daily living at a level consistent with disease state and treatment.
    * Identify health services and community resources available for managing changes in mobility.
    * Use assistive devices to aid or improve mobility.
    * Implement measures to prevent the complications of decreased mobility (e.g., pressure ulcers, pneumonia).

Figure 12-1. Standards Applicable to Physical Activity and Chronic Cancer-Related Conditions

---

(Continued on next page)

Standard IV. Planning
- Incorporate appropriate preventive, therapeutic, rehabilitative, and palliative nursing actions into each phase of the plan of care along the cancer trajectory.
- Develop the plan of care in collaboration with the patient, family, interdisciplinary cancer care team, and other healthcare professionals when possible.

Standard V. Implementation
- Use evidence-based research to guide implementation of interventions.

Standard VI. Evaluation
- Communicate the patient's response with the interdisciplinary cancer care team and other agencies involved in the healthcare continuum.

Figure 12-1. Standards Applicable to Physical Activity and Chronic Cancer-Related Conditions *(Continued)*

Note. From *Statement on the Scope and Standards of Oncology Nursing Practice: Generalist and Advanced Practice,* by J.M. Brant and R. Wickham (Eds.), 2013, Pittsburgh, PA: Oncology Nursing Society. Copyright 2013 by Oncology Nursing Society. Adapted with permission.

transport capacity is reduced as a result of functional or acquired causes (Zuther & Norton, 2013).

Lymphedema, an abnormal accumulation of protein-rich lymph fluid associated with either a malformed or malfunctioning lymphatic system, is an unfortunate result of cancer treatment for many cancer survivors. Mechanical insufficiency, also known as secondary lymphedema, is most often due to causes such as surgery, radiation, trauma, or infection and most frequently is experienced by cancer survivors (Lawenda, Mondry, & Johnstone, 2009). The stages of lymphedema are as follows (Zuther & Norton, 2013):

- Latency: No swelling
- Subclinical: Reduced transport capacity; normal tissue consistency
- Reversible: Edema is soft (pitting); no secondary tissue changes; elevation reduces swelling
- Spontaneously irreversible: Lymphostatic fibrosis; hardening of the tissue (no pitting); Stemmer sign–positive; frequent infections
- Lymphostatic elephantiasis: Extreme increase in volume and tissue texture with typical skin changes (papillomas, deep skinfolds, etc.); Stemmer sign–positive

An estimated three million individuals in the United States have been diagnosed with lymphedema; many of these individuals are cancer survivors (Zuther & Norton, 2013). The development of lymphedema in cancer survivorship usually is the result of lymphadenectomy during the staging and surgical treatment of cancers or from damage to superficial lymphatics or remaining lymph nodes by radiation therapy techniques. Malignancies that pose a risk for lymphedema include but are not limited to breast cancer, melanoma, genitourinary cancers, gynecologic cancers, colorectal cancers, head and neck cancers, and sarcoma.

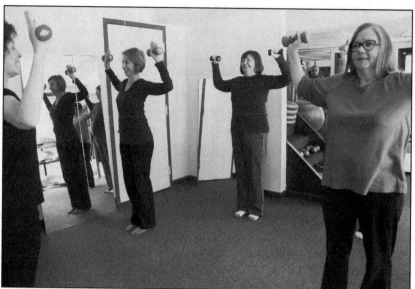

Strength and resistance endurance exercises are safe for cancer survivors experiencing lymphedema.

Ahmed, Schmitz, Prizment, and Folsom (2011) assessed risk factors and related arm symptoms in 1,287 breast cancer survivors in the Iowa Women's Health Study. They concluded that tumor stage, number of excised nodes, tumor-positive nodes, and adjuvant chemotherapy were cancer characteristics positively associated with lymphedema. In addition, they found greater baseline body mass index, greater waist and hip circumference, and lower levels of general health to be associated with lymphedema. Regarding upper extremity symptoms, higher numbers of excised nodes, axillary radiation, and lower baseline general health characteristics were positively associated with lymphedema. In a systematic review of 47 studies (7,779 cancer survivors) that examined the incidence of lymphedema as a consequence of cancer and cancer treatment techniques in non–breast cancer malignancies, the overall incidence of lymphedema was 15.5% (Cormier et al., 2010). The incidence varied by malignancy, location of node dissection, and treatment modalities used, with sarcoma (30%), melanoma of the lower extremity (28%), and gynecologic cancers (20%) having the highest incidence rates. They also identified an increased lymphedema risk for individuals undergoing pelvic dissections (22%) and radiation therapy (31%). Shaitelman et al. (2015) reassessed lymphedema incidence rates in breast cancer as a follow-up to the work by Lawenda et al. (2009) to include average, range, and pooled incidence rates. Their review of the literature revealed breast cancer–related lymphedema pooled incidence following sentinel lymph node biopsy to be 6.3% (average [avg.], 7%; range,

0%–23%) and 22.3% following axillary lymph node dissection (avg., 28%; range, 11%–57%). Additionally, Shaitelman et al. (2015) reported on lymphedema incidence in melanoma (avg., 6.1%; range, 0.6%–15%; pooled incidence, 4.1%), gynecologic cancers (avg., 25.1%; range, 2%–49%; pooled incidence, 27%), penile cancer (avg., 20.5%; range, 20%–21%; pooled incidence, 21%), bladder cancer (avg., 19%; range, 15%–23%; pooled incidence, 16%), prostate cancer (avg., 8%; range, 1%–18%; pooled incidence, 4%), and head and neck cancers (range, 0%–8%).

McNeely et al. (2012) and Stout et al. (2012) advocated for prospective surveillance models of care to provide early identification of deficits and standardized processes for routine measurements and structured care for breast cancer survivors at risk for the development of lymphedema. These measures have the potential to identify lymphedema early (when it can be more easily managed) as well as provide an overall cost savings within the healthcare system. Rehabilitation professionals with experience in lymphedema management should, therefore, be considered an integral part of the cancer treatment plan for all at-risk cancer survivors, as well as their long-term survivorship care plan, in order to support and treat conditions as they arise and restore functional mobility, activity participation, and quality of life.

A systematic review of 26 articles by Lasinski et al. (2012) found that complete decongestive therapy, as a bundled intervention of manual lymphatic drainage and compression bandaging, was effective in reducing lymphedema. Because exercise had long been considered potentially detrimental to patients at risk for lymphedema, Schmitz et al. (2009) designed the Physical Activity and Lymphedema Trial to examine this risk in a randomized fashion. Through the trial, they were able to successfully demonstrate the safety of slowly progressive weight lifting compared with no exercise; weight lifting did not result in increased incidence of lymphedema in breast cancer survivors at risk for lymphedema (Schmitz et al., 2010). However, the low intensity of the resistance training in the trial did not demonstrate a benefit to bone health by bone mineral density testing (Winters-Stone, Laudermilk, Woo, Brown, & Schmitz, 2014). While examining varied loads of resistance, Cormie et al. (2013) randomized 62 participants with breast cancer–related lymphedema (high-load resistance exercise [n = 22], low-load resistance exercise [n = 21], or usual care [n = 19]) for a period of three months and found no differences between groups in the extent of affected arm swelling or severity of symptoms. Kwan, Cohn, Armer, Stewart, and Cormier (2011) completed a systematic review of exercise in the management of lymphedema and found strong evidence on the safety of resis-

Resistance exercise is safe for cancer survivors experiencing lymphedema when properly prescribed. Consult with a lymphedema-certified physical or occupational therapist to select appropriate activities and exercises.

tance exercise without an increase in risk of lymphedema for patients with breast cancer.

Application to Oncology Nursing Practice

Self-Report and Lymphedema Screening Measures

1. Obtain your oncology center's lymphedema assessment protocol and review the questions you ask cancer survivors about the presence of lymphedema.
2. Assess for lymphedema at each clinic visit.
3. Determine if a referral to a lymphedema-certified physical therapist (PT) or occupational therapist (OT) is needed.

Self-Report and Physical Activity/Exercise Assessment

1. Assess current physical activity and exercise patterns using measures such as those described in Chapter 4.
2. Use the physical activity and exercise measures endorsed by your oncology center to measure activity. Assess cancer survivors' current physical activity and exercise program to note any relationship between the presence of lymphedema and level of physical activity in which the survivor is currently engaged.

Oncology Nursing Recommendations for Physical Activity and Exercise to Manage Lymphedema

1. Use any of the interviewing techniques discussed in Chapter 5 to determine survivors' readiness to incorporate physical activity and exercise into their lifestyle.
2. Teach survivors about the potential benefits of physical activity and exercise for lymphedema.
3. Refer to a lymphedema-certified PT or OT for lymphedema management with complete decongestive therapy, including manual lymphatic drainage, compression, exercise, and skin care. Cancer survivors with existing lymphedema who are interested in starting an exercise program should be referred for a PT or OT evaluation for assessment of compression needs and exercise prescription. They may require supervision and monitoring of lymphedema during the initial phase of the new activities and to ensure proper fit of appropriate compression garments.
4. Use the evidence presented in this chapter to create a patient education fact sheet for lymphedema and physical activity. Use the education materials provided by your oncology center. Assure survivors that an individual-

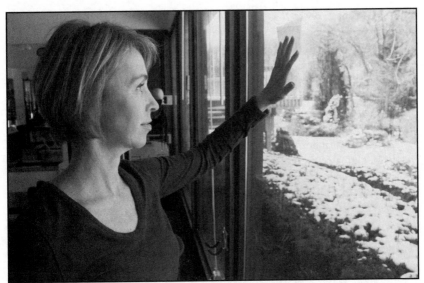

Reaching shoulder height or overhead during light housekeeping can be beneficial for shoulder range of motion and strengthening.

ized physical activity and exercise plan has been shown to be safe for help-ing with lymphedema management.

5. Encourage survivors to report to you any new or exacerbated symptoms after starting physical activity and exercise in order to discuss ways to reduce these symptoms.

6. Collaborate with cancer survivors to select physical activities and exer-cises they enjoy and are able to perform regularly and safely. Use check-lists offered by your oncology center or the lists provided in Chapters 1 and 4.

7. Select a method for tracking physical activity and lymphedema. Ask survi-vors to bring the tracking program with them on their next visit.

Oncology Nursing Evaluation of Health Outcomes

1. Evaluate cancer survivors' adherence to the lymphedema management program and note any improvements in or worsening of the lymph-edema.

2. Revise the physical activity and exercise plans as needed. Adjust the fre-quency, intensity, time, and type of activities to meet the needs of cancer survivors.

3. Follow up with referrals for lymphedema evaluation with a PT or OT certified in lymphedema management as advised by your oncology cen-ter.

Cancer Cachexia

An unfortunate and debilitating potential side effect in oncology is cancer cachexia or anorexia-cachexia syndrome, which results in wasting of both adipose and skeletal muscle tissue. Fearon et al. (2011) described cachexia as "a multifactorial syndrome defined by an ongoing loss of skeletal muscle mass (with or without loss of fat mass) that cannot be fully reversed by conventional nutritional support and leads to progressive functional impairment" (p. 489). The criteria for cachexia was determined by Fearon et al. (2011) and includes weight loss greater than 5%; weight loss greater than 2% in individuals with a body mass index under 20; or sarcopenia (< 7.26 kg/m² for men; < 5.45 kg/m² for women). In addition to anorexia and loss of adipose and skeletal muscle tissue, characteristics of cancer cachexia also often include early satiety and weakness.

Incidence rate estimates for cachexia are as high as 50% for all cancer survivors, with prevalence rates rising to as high as 86% within two weeks of death (Vaughan, Martin, & Lewandowski, 2013). In their international consensus, Fearon et al. (2011) suggested three clinical stages of cachexia: precachexia, cachexia, and refractory cachexia. The criteria for precachexia include weight loss of 5% or greater and/or anorexia. The criteria for refractory cachexia include active catabolism, where management of weight loss is no longer possible or appropriate, low performance status (i.e., World Health Organization score of 3 or 4), and life expectancy of less than three months (Fearon et al., 2011).

No definitive or curative therapies for cancer cachexia currently exist; treatment strategies target the underlying malignancy first. Weakness associated with muscle atrophy is theorized to be caused by a reduction in protein synthesis or an increase in protein degradation (Del Fabbro, Inui, & Strasser, 2012). Despite the potential benefits of physical activity to address muscle atrophy, a systematic review of exercise for cancer cachexia in adults by Grande et al. (2014) found insufficient evidence to determine safety and effectiveness.

Application to Oncology Nursing Practice

Self-Report and Cachexia Screening Measures

1. Assess for cachexia using the diagnostic and clinical staging criteria mentioned in this chapter.
2. Obtain your oncology center's current guidelines for measuring cachexia and compare your center's practice with the criteria listed in this chapter.
3. Determine if a referral for nutrition services is needed based on the self-assessment and screening.

Self-Report and Physical Activity/Exercise Assessment

1. Assess current physical activity and exercise patterns using measures such as those described in Chapter 4. Use the physical activity and exercise measures endorsed by your oncology center to measure activity. Assessing cancer survivors' current physical activity and exercise program will help you understand the level of physical activity in which they are currently engaged.
2. Evaluate the relationship between cancer survivors' physical activity and cachexia. Assess the frequency, intensity, time, and type of activities being performed. Are the activities too strenuous for the cancer survivor? Is the survivor too cachexic to perform activities of daily living, leading to additional loss of muscle mass?
3. Determine if a consultation with a PT or OT is indicated if functional mobility impairments are observed or if assistive devices may be needed for ambulation or adaptive equipment for activities of daily living. A home safety assessment and caregiver training regarding transfer techniques, fall risk reduction, and proper patient positioning may be beneficial.

Oncology Nursing Recommendations for Physical Activity and Exercise for Cachexia

1. Use any of the interviewing techniques discussed in Chapter 5 to determine cancer survivors' readiness to incorporate physical activity or exercise into their lifestyle.
2. Teach survivors about the benefits of physical activity to improve muscle mass. Regarding the role of exercise in cachexia, a systematic review by Grande et al. (2014) revealed insufficient evidence to determine the safety and effectiveness of exercise for patients with cancer cachexia. However, when prescribed by a PT for a medically stable individual motivated to participate, physical activity is targeted at maintaining functional strength for activities of daily living and balance for fall risk reduction. Light resistance exercise, individually prescribed by a PT, may be used to help to maintain muscle mass. Short-duration aerobic activity, such as an interval walking program, may help to maintain cardiovascular capacity and release endorphins to improve the sense of well-being. Prolonged high-intensity aerobic activities or heavy resistance training, which would in turn require excessive caloric expenditure, should be discouraged.
3. Use the evidence presented in this chapter to create a patient education fact sheet. Use the education materials provided by your oncology center. Assure cancer survivors that individualized physical activity and exercise plans have been shown to be safe for cancer survivors with cachexia.

4. Collaborate with survivors to select physical activities and exercises they enjoy and are able to perform regularly and safely. Use checklists offered by your oncology center or the lists provided in Chapter 4. Be sure to do the following when selecting activities:
   - Try to avoid activities that would cause skin shearing, particularly in those who are debilitated. In the instance of lost subcutaneous fat over bony prominences, such as with cachexia, the risk of pressure ulcers is increased. In a postmortem case-control study by Pueschel, Heinemann, Krause, Anders, and von Renteln-Kruse (2005), cachexia was noted in 66% of older adult patients with grades 3 and 4 decubitus ulcers. The estimated prevalence rate of pressure ulcers in palliative care cases is 22.9%, with an incidence rate of 6.7% (Hendrichova et al., 2010). An estimated 2.5 million pressure ulcer cases are reported in the United States each year, with a total annual cost of $11 billion (Cushing & Phillips, 2013). Considering these facts, focused attention should be placed on preventive strategies. In the oncology patient population, comprehensive pressure ulcer prevention strategies should include risk assessment, skin care, offloading, and nutrition (Lyder, 2006).
   - Immobility also places cancer survivors at greater risk. Care should be given to ensure proper positioning to protect the skin (e.g., frequently changing positions, using alternating pressure mattresses, reducing shear forces during transfers, maximizing activity level, performing proper skin care, using seating systems incorporating gel, air, or foam).
5. Select a method for tracking physical activity and weight/nutrition patterns. Ask cancer survivors to bring the tracking program with them on their next visit.

Oncology Nursing Evaluation of Health Outcomes

1. Evaluate cancer survivors' adherence to their recommended physical activity/exercise plan by discussing their self-report outcomes.
2. Evaluate these outcomes to the plan adherence and survivors' weight and body mass. Note any improvements in or worsening of their health status.
3. Revise the physical activity and exercise plans as needed. Adjust the frequency, intensity, time, and type of activities to meet patients' needs.
4. Follow up with referrals for physical or occupational therapy and nutrition services as required by your oncology center.

Bone Loss and Fracture Risk

Cancer treatment–related side effects, such as those caused by the use of chemotherapy agents, radiation therapy, endocrine therapy, and corticosteroids, can predispose cancer survivors to bone loss. In hormone-associated cancers, surgical- and chemical-induced (via antiestrogen agents) menopause for the purpose of breast cancer treatment in females and androgen deprivation therapy (ADT) use in prostate cancer can result in osteopenia or osteoporosis in cancer survivors. Melton et al. (2012) studied a population-based historical cohort study of 608 invasive breast cancer survivors and found their overall fracture risk was increased 1.8-fold. Taylor, Canfield, and Du (2009) found that prostate cancer survivors who received ADT had an increased overall fracture risk of 23% when compared to men who did not receive ADT. Even hormone-naïve prostate cancer survivors were found to have a rate of osteoporosis ranging from 4%–38% in a meta-analysis by Lassemillante, Doi, Hooper, Prins, and Wright (2015). The authors also observed that patients with more advanced disease had a higher prevalence of osteoporosis. In 7,620 patients who underwent a hematopoietic stem cell transplantation, fracture incidence in patients aged 45–64 years was found to be eight times greater in female patients and seven to nine times greater in male patients than compared to the general U.S. population (Pundole, Barbo, Lin, Champlin, & Lu, 2015).

Radiation therapy techniques have also been shown to have detrimental effects on the bone health of cancer survivors. Ugurluer, Akbas, Arpaci, Ozcan, and Serin (2014) retrospectively reviewed the incidence of pelvic bone complications via magnetic resonance imaging testing following pelvic radiation in 345 cancer survivors and found the following: pelvic insufficiency fracture (13.9%, with a total of 64 lesions); radiation osteitis (4.1%, with a total of 13 lesions); and avascular necrosis of the femoral head (0.8%). Uezono et al. (2013) studied the incidence of pelvic insufficiency fracture in 126 patients with a history of uterine cancer who were treated with definitive radiation therapy. A review by Kim et al. (2012) of the incidence of sacral fractures after chemoradiation for locally advanced rectal carcinoma in 582 patients demonstrated a 7.1% (35 of 492) incidence of fracture (median follow-up time of 3.5 years). According to Elliott et al. (2011), the use of pelvic three-dimensional conformal external beam radiation therapy in men with prostate cancer was associated with a 76% increased risk of hip fracture. Regarding radiation therapy to the chest, particularly brachytherapy, an increased risk for rib fracture in breast cancer survivors has been documented (Smith et al., 2012).

The National Comprehensive Cancer Network® (NCCN®) recommends routine screening of bone health for at-risk patients throughout survivorship in the *NCCN Task Force Report: Bone Health in Cancer Care* (Gralow et al., 2013). On behalf of the American Society of Clinical Oncology, Van Poznak (2015) recommended counseling on calcium intake with vitamin D, exercise, behavior modifications (e.g., limiting tobacco and alcohol consumption), monitoring for fall risk, and educating about the effects of steroids. Pharmacologic management approved by the U.S. Food and Drug Administration, such as bisphosphonates, monoclonal antibodies, and hormonal therapies, should be discussed with the medical provider (Van Poznak, 2015). In a randomized controlled trial of 106 women with early-stage breast cancer, women in the moderate-intensity resistance and impact training program preserved bone mineral density (in grams per square centimeter) at the lumbar (L) spine (L1–L4) (0.47% vs. –2.13%; p = 0.001) compared to controls who performed low-intensity stretching (Winters-Stone et al., 2014). However, a systematic review of prostate cancer survivors provided inconclusive evidence concerning the effect of resistance exercise on bone mineral density (Hasenoehrl et al., 2015).

Application to Oncology Nursing Practice

Self-Report and Screening Measures

1. Assess for bone loss in at-risk cancer survivors at intervals determined by your oncology center. Obtain the survivor's medication list and evaluate the list for bisphosphonates, monoclonal antibodies, hormonal therapies, or radiation therapy.
2. Obtain your oncology center's current guidelines for when and how bone loss is measured in cancer survivors.
3. Determine if a referral for physical therapy is needed based on the self-assessment and screening.

Self-Report and Physical Activity/Exercise Assessment

1. Assess current physical activity and exercise patterns using measures such as those described in Chapter 4. Use the physical activity and exercise measures endorsed by your oncology center to measure activity.
2. Evaluate the relationship between the cancer survivors' physical activity and bone health. Assess the frequency, intensity, time, and type of activities. Do the activities include strength and conditioning for the upper and lower body, as well as activities that include balance?
3. Determine if a consultation to a PT or OT is indicated if functional mobility impairments are observed or if the cancer survivor presents with postural deviations.

Oncology Nursing Recommendations for Physical Activity and Exercise for Bone Loss

1. Use any of the interviewing techniques discussed in Chapter 5 to determine survivors' readiness to incorporate physical activity and/or exercise into their lifestyle.
2. Teach cancer survivors about the benefits of physical activity to improve muscle mass.
3. Collaborate with survivors to select physical activities and exercises they enjoy and are able to perform regularly and safely. Use checklists offered by

your oncology center or the lists provided in Chapter 4. Safe lifting techniques and fall risk prevention strategies should be developed with a PT for individuals with a diagnosis of osteopenia or osteoporosis. Resistance and weight-bearing exercises should be encouraged for survivors at risk for or with a confirmed diagnosis of bone loss. Table 12-1 outlines a common-sense approach to physical activities and exercises for people at risk for fractures.

4. Select a method for tracking physical activity and exercise. Ask survivors to bring the tracking program with them on their next visit.

Oncology Nursing Evaluation of Health Outcomes

1. Evaluate survivors' adherence to the recommended physical activity/exercise plan by discussing their self-report outcomes.

Table 12-1. Common-Sense Approach to Physical Activity and Exercise for People at Risk for Fractures

Recommendation	Rationale
Walk on even, dry surfaces, such as a track, gym floor, etc.	Helps to prevent slippage and may reduce the risk of subsequent falls
Participate in resistance exercises of larger muscle groups.	Promotes muscle strength to maintain muscle mass and support bones
Participate in weight-bearing exercises (upper and lower body); for example, upper body: push hands against wall; lower body: stand and walk. May use hiking poles bilaterally for ambulation to encourage light weight-bearing on the upper extremities.	Promotes bone loading to increase bone mineral density
Wear proper-fitting shoes and clothing appropriate for activity (e.g., well-fitted gloves for gardening, shoes for walking or biking).	Prevents slippage and potential injury
Participate in activities that promote balance, such as standing on one leg and holding on to the wall or horizontal railing. Use handrails and walls for balance support when active as needed for safety.	Promotes proprioception and balance
Monitor self for proper spinal posture in sitting, standing, and while performing activities of daily living.	Helps reduce pressure on the spinal column and discourages the progression of postural deviations (e.g., forward head, excessive thoracic kyphosis)

2. Evaluate these outcomes to the plan adherence.
3. Revise the physical activity and exercise plans as needed. Adjust the frequency, intensity, time, and type of activities to meet survivors' needs.
4. Follow up with a referral for physical therapy as required by your oncology center.

Cancer-Related Emergencies

Most oncology clinicians are familiar with the potential risk for rare metabolic, cardiovascular, neurologic, infectious, hematologic, and respiratory emergencies in the cancer survivors in their care. Lewis, Hendrickson, and Moynihan (2011) reviewed the pathophysiology, presentation, diagnosis, and treatment of oncologic emergencies and provided an excellent summary as a reminder of their incidence. When supervising patients receiving physical activity as part of their treatment plan, oncology nurses should be aware of the typical signs and symptoms of oncologic emergencies and know when to refer cancer survivors for further evaluation and intervention. Cancer survivors and caregivers also should be educated about the signs and symptoms of the emergencies of which they are at greatest risk as well as the proper steps to take, whom to contact, and where to go if symptoms arise. Basic safety precautions of keeping a phone nearby, staying hydrated, and avoiding overexertion are always helpful reminders.

Summary

Although cancer survivors may present with several special considerations that the oncology clinician must be aware of and accommodate for, they also have many similarities with the general population. Despite many years of national recommendations for proper dietary intake and adequate physical activity as standard of cancer in oncology (Rock et al., 2012), cancer survivors often face the same issues as the average adult in the United States including overweight and obesity, lack of regular physical activity, poor dietary intake, and tobacco use. Oncology nurses need to consider these commonalities before adding the complexities of physical activity and exercise recommendations with their cancer diagnoses and treatment- and disease-related side effects.

Cancer survivors often struggle with impairments associated with their cancer diagnosis and treatment that require special attention from their oncology nurses. With proper awareness and accommodations, even the most challenging cases can be safely handled. Creating an interprofessional team that can effectively address needs comprehensively can also help to ensure the best possible outcome for individual cancer survivors. Future directions in the rapidly emerging field of oncology rehabilitation will include innovative interprofessional collaborations and coordinated research efforts, including large-scale prospective cohort studies that sufficiently describe their rehabilitation needs through the continuum of the survivorship experience to establish both a robust framework to support future investigation and shared initiatives (Stubblefield et al., 2013).

Case Study

D.J., a 51-year-old woman, is an avid exerciser who works out five to six days per week. She is married and has one daughter. D.J. previously worked in the front office of a neurosurgery practice. She occasionally drinks wine and is dedicated to fitness. One day while riding her bike, D.J. fell and hit her head, resulting in headaches and decreased energy. She did not seek medical evaluation at that time. In November, she developed a "cold" with a persistent cough and hoarseness. A chest x-ray and computed tomography (CT) scan of her chest revealed a 2.8 × 1.7 cm mass in the right paratracheal region. A CT scan of her brain was negative. A CT of her abdomen revealed multiple space-occupying lesions in the liver. A liver biopsy revealed small-cell lung carcinoma. D.J. experiences dyspnea on exertion, diminished appetite, and a six-pound weight loss. She has pain in her right shoulder and chest at 3/10 on the numeric pain rating scale. D.J. has stopped exercising completely.

The plan of care is no surgery and chemotherapy every 21 days, with reassessment after six cycles.

Medical History
• Breast augmentation
• Anterior cruciate ligament and meniscus repair
• Tubal ligation

Medications
• Carboplatin
• Etoposide

What would be best to help support D.J.?
  Services provided include
• Nutrition consultation
• Social services consultation for D.J. and her husband for adjustment to illness and work-related leave of absence
• Physical therapist patient education regarding fitness level and exercise prescription and safety
• Referral to the cancer center's exercise program with transition to an independent, gym-based exercise program (including cycling and yoga)
• Massage and Reiki during chemotherapy

(Case study continues in Chapter 13)

References

Ahmed, R.L., Schmitz, K.H., Prizment, A.E., & Folsom, A.R. (2011). Risk factors for lymphedema in breast cancer survivors, the Iowa Women's Health Study. *Breast Cancer Research and Treatment, 130,* 981–991. doi:10.1007/s10549-011-1667-z

Brant, J.M., & Wickham, R. (Eds.). (2013). *Statement on the scope and standards of oncology nursing practice: Generalist and advanced practice.* Pittsburgh, PA: Oncology Nursing Society.

Cormie, P., Pumpa, K., Galvão, D.A., Turner, E., Spry, N., Saunders, C., ... Newton, R.U. (2013). Is it safe and efficacious for women with lymphedema secondary to breast cancer to lift heavy weights during exercise: A randomised controlled trial. *Journal of Cancer Survivorship, 7,* 413–424. doi:10.1007/s11764-013-0284-8

Cormier, J.N., Askew, R.L., Mungovan, K.S., Xing, Y., Ross, M.I., & Armer, J.M. (2010). Lymphedema beyond breast cancer: A systematic review and meta-analysis of cancer-related secondary lymphedema. *Cancer, 116,* 5138–5149. doi:10.1002/cncr.25458

Cushing, C.A., & Phillips, L.G. (2013). Evidence-based medicine: Pressure sores. *Plastic and Reconstructive Surgery, 132,* 1720–1732. doi:10.1097/PRS.0b013e3182a808ba

Del Fabbro, E., Inui, A., & Strasser, F. (2012). *Cancer cachexia.* New York, NY: Springer Healthcare.

Elliott, S.P., Jarosek, S.L., Alanee, S.R., Konety, B.R., Dusenbery, K.E., & Virnig, B.A. (2011). Three-dimensional external beam radiotherapy for prostate cancer increases the risk of hip fracture. *Cancer, 117,* 4557–4565. doi:10.1002/cncr.25994

Fearon, K., Strasser, F., Anker, S.D., Bosaeus, I., Bruera, E., Fainsinger, R.L., ... Baracos, V.E. (2011). Definition and classification of cancer cachexia: An international consensus. *Lancet Oncology, 12,* 489–495. doi:10.1016/S1470-2045(10)70218-7

Gralow, J.R., Biermann, J.S., Farooki, A., Fornier, M.N., Gagel, R.F., Kumar, R., ... Van Poznak, C.H. (2013). NCCN Task Force report: Bone health in cancer care. *Journal of the National Comprehensive Cancer Network, 11*(Suppl. 3), S1–S51. Retrieved from https://www.nccn.org/JNCCN/supplements/PDF/bone_health_cancer_care_tf.pdf

Grande, A.J., Silva, V., Riera, R., Medeiros, A., Vitoriano, S.G.P., Peccin, M.S., & Maddocks, M. (2014). Exercise for cancer cachexia in adults. *Cochrane Database of Systematic Reviews, 2014*(11). doi:10.1002/14651858.CD010804.pub2

Hasenoehrl, T., Keilani, M., Komanadj, T.S., Mickel, M., Margreiter, M., Marhold, M., & Crevenna, R. (2015). The effects of resistance exercise on physical performance and health-related quality of life in prostate cancer patients: A systematic review. *Supportive Care in Cancer, 23,* 2479–2497. doi:10.1007/s00520-015-2782-x

Hendrichova, I., Castelli, M., Mastroianni, C., Piredda, M., Mirabella, F., Surdo, L., ... Casale, G. (2010). Pressure ulcers in cancer palliative care patients. *Palliative Medicine, 24,* 669–673. doi:10.1177/0269216310376119

Kim, H.J., Boland, P.J., Meredith, D.S., Lis, E., Zhang, Z., Shi, W., ... Goodman, K.A. (2012). Fractures of the sacrum after chemoradiation for rectal carcinoma: Incidence, risk factors, and radiographic evaluation. *International Journal of Radiation Oncology, Biology, Physics, 84,* 694–699. doi:10.1016/j.ijrobp.2012.01.021

Kwan, M.L., Cohn, J.C., Armer, J.M., Stewart, B.R., & Cormier, J.N. (2011). Exercise in patients with lymphedema: A systematic review of the contemporary literature. *Journal of Cancer Survivorship, 5,* 320–336. doi:10.1007/s11764-011-0203-9

Lasinski, B.B., Thrift, K.M., Squire, D., Austin, M.K., Smith, K.M., Wanchai, A., ... Armer, J.M. (2012). A systematic review of the evidence for complete decongestive therapy in the treatment of lymphedema from 2004 to 2011. *PM&R, 4,* 580–601. doi:10.1016/j.pmrj.2012.05.003

Lassemillante, A.-C., Doi, S.A., Hooper, J.D., Prins, J.B., & Wright, O.R. (2015). Prevalence of osteoporosis in prostate cancer survivors II: A meta-analysis of men not on androgen deprivation therapy. *Endocrine, 50,* 344–354. doi:10.1007/s12020-015-0536-7

Lawenda, B.D., Mondry, T.E., & Johnstone, P.A. (2009). Lymphedema: A primer on the identification and management of a chronic condition in oncologic treatment. *CA: A Cancer Journal for Clinicians, 59,* 8–24. doi:10.3322/caac.20001

Lewis, M.A., Hendrickson, A.W., & Moynihan, T.J. (2011). Oncologic emergencies: Pathophysiology, presentation, diagnosis, and treatment. *CA: A Cancer Journal for Clinicians, 61,* 287–314. doi:10.3322/caac.20124

Lyder, C.H. (2006). Assessing risk and preventing pressure ulcers in patients with cancer. *Seminars in Oncology Nursing, 22,* 178–184. doi:10.1016/j.soncn.2006.04.002

McNeely, M.L., Binkley, J.M., Pusic, A.L., Campbell, K.L., Gabram, S., & Soballe, P.W. (2012). A prospective model of care for breast cancer rehabilitation: Postoperative and postreconstructive issues. *Cancer, 118*(Suppl. 8), 2226–2236. doi:10.1002/cncr.27468

Melton, L.J., Hartmann, L.C., Achenbach, S.J., Atkinson, E.J., Therneau, T.M., & Khosla, S. (2012). Fracture risk in women with breast cancer: A population-based study. *Journal of Bone and Mineral Research, 27,* 1196–1205. doi:10.1002/jbmr.1556

Pueschel, K., Heinemann, A., Krause, T., Anders, S., & von Renteln-Kruse, W. (2005). High-grade decubitus ulcers in the elderly: A postmortem case-control study of risk factors. *Forensic Science, Medicine, and Pathology, 1,* 193–196. doi:10.1385/FSMP:1:3:193

Pundole, X.N., Barbo, A.G., Lin, H., Champlin, R.E., & Lu, H. (2015). Increased incidence of fractures in recipients of hematopoietic stem-cell transplantation. *Journal of Clinical Oncology, 33,* 1364–1370. doi:10.1200/JCO.2014.57.8195

Rock, C.L., Doyle, C., Demark-Wahnefried, W., Meyerhardt, J., Courneya, K.S., Schwartz, A.L., ... Gansler, T. (2012). Nutrition and physical activity guidelines for cancer survivors. *CA: A Cancer Journal for Clinicians, 62,* 243–274. doi:10.3322/caac.21142

Schmitz, K.H., Ahmed, R.L., Troxel, A.B., Cheville, A., Lewis-Grant, L., Smith, R., ... Chittams, J. (2010). Weight lifting for women at risk for breast cancer–related lymphedema: A randomized trial. *JAMA, 304,* 2699–2705. doi:10.1001/jama.2010.1837

Schmitz, K.H., Troxel, A.B., Cheville, A., Grant, L.L., Bryan, C.J., Gross, C.R., ... Ahmed, R.L. (2009). Physical activity and lymphedema (the PAL trial): Assessing the safety of progressive strength training in breast cancer survivors. *Contemporary Clinical Trials, 30,* 233–245. doi:10.1016/j.cct.2009.01.001

Shaitelman, S.F., Cromwell, K.D., Rasmussen, J.C., Stout, N.L., Armer, J.M., Lasinski, B.B., & Cormier, J.N. (2015). Recent progress in the treatment and prevention of cancer-related lymphedema. *CA: A Cancer Journal for Clinicians, 65,* 55–81. doi:10.3322/caac.21253

Smith, G.L., Xu, Y., Buchholz, T.A., Giordano, S.H., Jiang, J., Shih, Y.-C., & Smith, B.D. (2012). Association between treatment with brachytherapy vs whole-breast irradiation and subsequent mastectomy, complications, and survival among older women with invasive breast cancer. *JAMA, 307,* 1827–1837. doi:10.1001/jama.2012.3481

Stout, N.L., Pfalzer, L.A., Springer, B., Levy, E., McGarvey, C.L., Danoff, J.V., ... Soballe, P.W. (2012). Breast cancer–related lymphedema: Comparing direct costs of a prospective surveillance model and a traditional model of care. *Physical Therapy, 92,* 152–163. doi:10.2522/ptj.20100167

Stubblefield, M.D., Hubbard, G., Cheville, A., Koch, U., Schmitz, K.H., & Dalton, S.O. (2013). Current perspectives and emerging issues on cancer rehabilitation. *Cancer, 119*(Suppl. 11), 2170–2178. doi:10.1002/cncr.28059

Taylor, L.G., Canfield, S.E., & Du, X.L. (2009). Review of major adverse effects of androgen-deprivation therapy in men with prostate cancer. *Cancer, 115,* 2388–2399. doi:10.1002/cncr.24283

Uezono, H., Tsujino, K., Moriki, K., Nagano, F., Ota, Y., Sasaki, R., & Soejima, T. (2013). Pelvic insufficiency fracture after definitive radiotherapy for uterine cervical cancer: Retrospective analysis of risk factors. *Journal of Radiation Research, 54,* 1102–1109. doi:10.1093/jrr/rrt055

Ugurluer, G., Akbas, T., Arpaci, T., Ozcan, N., & Serin, M. (2014). Bone complications after pelvic radiation therapy: Evaluation with MRI. *Journal of Medical Imaging and Radiation Oncology, 58,* 334–340. doi:10.1111/1754-9485.12176

Van Poznak, C.H. (2015). Bone health in adults treated with endocrine therapy for early breast or prostate cancer. *American Society of Clinical Oncology Educational Book*. Retrieved from http://meetinglibrary.asco.org/content/11500567-156

Vaughan, V.C., Martin, P., & Lewandowski, P.A. (2013). Cancer cachexia: Impact, mechanisms, and emerging treatments. *Journal of Cachexia, Sarcopenia and Muscle, 4,* 95–109. doi:10.1007/s13539-012-0087-1

Winters-Stone, K.M., Laudermilk, M., Woo, K., Brown, J.C., & Schmitz, K.H. (2014). Influence of weight training on skeletal health of breast cancer survivors with or at risk for breast cancer–related lymphedema. *Journal of Cancer Survivorship, 8,* 260–268. doi:10.1007/s11764-013-0337-z

Zuther, J.E., & Norton, S. (2013). *Lymphedema management: The comprehensive guide for practitioners* (3rd ed.). New York, NY: Thieme Medical Publishers.

CHAPTER 13

Physical Activity for Metastatic and End-of-Life Conditions

Amy J. Litterini, PT, DPT

Introduction

Palliative rehabilitation emphasizes the preservation of quality of life through the maintenance of individual control and mobility, even in the face of progressive disease in patients who are terminally ill. Palliative rehabilitation measures should focus on maintaining patients' dignity and personhood through the provision of holistic care (Krishna, Yong, & Koh, 2014).

Dietz (1981) articulated the model for the role of oncology rehabilitation throughout the continuum of cancer care. This model ranges in scope and intensity of intervention from the preventive phase for predictable conditions through the palliative phase for irreversible conditions. This chapter focuses on the role of physical activity in people with metastatic cancer and facing end-of-life decisions. This chapter's content is supported in the Oncology Nursing Society's *Statement on the Scope and Standards of Oncology Nursing Practice: Generalist and Advanced Practice* (Brant & Wickham, 2013) (see Figure 12-1 in Chapter 12 for relevant standards).

Metastatic Disease

Cancer survivors with metastatic disease often experience a multitude of distressing symptoms, and some may not always be adequately addressed. Cheville, Troxel, Basford, and Kornblith (2008) assessed physical impairments in 163 community-dwelling patients with metastatic breast cancer. The majority presented with more than three impairments, 92% (482 of 530) required rehabilitation, and only 30% received an intervention.

Ruijs, Kerkhof, van der Wal, and Onwuteaka-Philipsen (2013) followed 77 patients receiving palliative care who had a six-month prognosis. They found that weakness was the most prevalent unbearable symptom (57%). Decreased functional mobility in patients with advanced cancer, as well as subsequent falls, decubitus ulcers, weakness, fatigue, and decreased ability to perform activities of daily living, can lead to additional pain and decreased quality of life, increased caregiver demand, and increased costs to the healthcare system.

Physical activity has become an accepted and more readily available option for long-term cancer survivors in general, as well as for those recently treated with curative intent. In a systematic review by Mishra et al. (2012), 40 randomized controlled trials with 3,694 patients demonstrated beneficial effects of physical activity for cancer survivors. The benefits included health-related quality of life and cancer-specific concerns (e.g., lessened fatigue, pain, and anxiety; improved emotional well-being). For cancer survivors with metastatic disease, a physically active approach not only has the potential to help with symptom management but also can provide patient empowerment and allow for functional independence for as long as feasibly possible.

A relatively small but growing number of studies suggest that exercise provides benefit to patients with advanced cancer. A systematic review by Beaton et al. (2009) examined eight studies of exercise interventions in patients with metastatic cancer. Based on consistent results from three randomized controlled trials, the authors determined that exercise interventions improve quality of life. Payne, Larkin, McIlfatrick, Dunwoody, and Gracey (2013) published a systematic review of five studies on exercise and/or nutrition interventions in advanced non-small cell lung cancer. In addition, beneficial effects on physical strength and functional performance were documented in the two exercise-only studies (N = 54) (Quist et al., 2012; Temel et al., 2009).

Lowe, Watanabe, Baracos, and Courneya (2010) assessed the physical activity interests and preferences of patients with cancer receiving palliative care and found the majority wanted to participate. Home-based exercise included walking programs and was preferred over other options. In a study with 66 adults diagnosed with stage IV colon or lung cancer, Cheville et al. (2013) established the feasibility of Rapid Easy Strength Training (REST). The trial consisted of two randomized groups; participants were either in the intervention group, an eight-week home-based exercise protocol and a monitored walking program, or the usual care group. Of those completing the protocol (intervention group: 26 of 33, usual care group: 30 of 33), the intervention group reported improved mobility (p = 0.01), fatigue (p = 0.02), and sleep quality (p = 0.05) when compared to usual care. The protocol was well tolerated, demonstrated a low dropout rate of 6%, and resulted in no adverse events.

Litterini and Fieler (2008) studied 200 participants with stages I–IV cancer (142 female, 58 male) during a physical therapist–prescribed strength, cardiovascular, and flexibility program twice weekly for 10 weeks at a hospital-based health club. The outcome measures were fatigue, lower extremity and hand grip strength, and quality of life. Of the 42 patients with stage IV cancer (22 female, 20 male), 26 (62%) completed the protocol and had statistically significant improvements in lower extremity strength (p = 0.03), quality of life (p = 0.03), and physical functioning (p = 0.05). Litterini, Fieler, Cavanaugh, and Lee (2013) compared the effects of cardiovascular and resistance training on functional mobility, fatigue, and pain following a 10-week supervised exercise program for 66 patients with end-stage cancer (terminal stage of all malignancies, 30 male, 36 female). Fifty-two patients (78.8%) completed the study, with outcomes including a significant increase in functional mobility (p < 0.001), increased gait speed (p = 0.001), and reduced fatigue (p = 0.05).

A quick assessment of gait speed in meters per second (m/sec) over a defined distance, such as four meters, with two meters each for acceleration and deceleration, can be an easy way to monitor for functional decline over time in cancer survivors in inpatient, outpatient, or home care settings (see Figure 13-1). In a pooled analysis of nine cohort studies with individual data from 34,485 community-dwelling adults aged 65 years or older, Studenski et al. (2011) determined gait speed was associated with survival in all studies (pooled hazard ratio per 0.1 m/sec, 0.88; 95% confidence interval [0.87–0.90]; p < 0.001). Increased survival was noted across the full range of gait speeds, with significant increments per 0.1 m/sec. With such a sensitive measure, subtle declines could potentially be identified over time with this patient population. This could be established as an indicator for referrals for rehabilitation interventions (e.g., a documented reduction of gait speed of 0.1 m/sec in an outpatient setting).

Due to the paucity of published research, few clinical guidelines exist to inform clinicians' decision making in individuals with advanced cancer. The most recently updated American Cancer Society physical activity guidelines for cancer survivorship stopped short of providing specific recommendations for

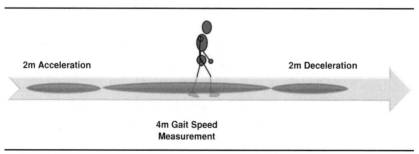

Figure 13-1. Measurement of Gait Speed

patients with advanced cancer due to insufficient data (Rock et al., 2012). In the National Comprehensive Cancer Network® (2016) guidelines, physical activity is recommended throughout all phases of cancer survivorship (see Table 13-1). Figure 13-2 provides a basic framework for exercise prescription for individuals with advanced cancer.

Skeletal Metastases

Skeletal metastases are a common occurrence in advanced cancers. The most common site of skeletal metastases is the axial skeleton, which includes the skull, rib cage, and spinal column (Coleman, 2006). Skeletal lesions can be osteolytic, osteoblastic, or mixed lytic and blastic. Osteolytic lesions are most common in lung and breast cancers, with osteoclast cell proliferation resulting in weak, porous bone. Osteoblastic lesions are most common in prostate cancer, with osteoblast cell proliferation resulting in thickened areas of bone tumor cells.

Cancer pain due to bone metastases is most effectively treated with external beam radiation therapy (Lutz et al., 2011). Radiation can provide significant

Table 13-1. Clinical Guidelines for Metastatic and End-of-Life Conditions

Phase of Survivorship	Nonpharmacologic Interventions
Patients on active treatment	• Consider starting and maintaining an exercise program, as appropriate per healthcare provider, of both endurance (walking, jogging, swimming) and resistance (light weights) exercises. • Consider referral to rehabilitation (physical therapy, occupational therapy, physical medicine). • When determining level of activity, special considerations include bone metastases, thrombocytopenia, anemia, fever or active infection, and limitations caused by metastases or other comorbid illnesses.
Patients after treatment	• Maintain optimal level of physical activity. • Consider initiation of exercise program of both endurance and resistance exercises. • Consider referral to rehabilitation (physical therapy, occupational therapy, physical medicine). • Exercise caution regarding late effects of treatment (e.g., cardiomyopathy).
Patients at the end of life	• Optimize level of physical activity with careful consideration of the following constraints: bone metastases, thrombocytopenia, anemia, fever, or active infection. • Assess safety issues (i.e., risk of falls, stability).

Note. Based on information from National Comprehensive Cancer Network, 2016.

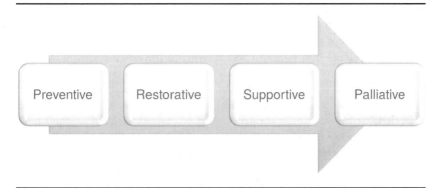

Figure 13-2. Phases of Oncology Rehabilitation

Note. Based on information from Dietz, 1981.

palliation of pain resulting from skeletal metastases in 50%–80% of patients. Up to one-third of patients experience complete pain relief in the treatment area (Chow, Harris, Fan, Tsao, & Sze, 2007).

Widespread bone metastasis also can lead to significant functional deficits, reduced independence, and diminished quality of life. In the instance of high-risk impending fracture, treatment may include prophylactic surgical fixation prior to irradiation. Mirels (2003) created a four-item scoring system that included the following variables:
• Degree of pain being experienced (mild, moderate, severe)
• Location of the lesion (upper limb, lower limb, peritrochanter)
• Type of lesion (lytic, blastic, mixed)
• Degree of cortex taken up by the lesion (less than 1/3, 1/3–2/3, greater than 2/3)

Mirels' criteria and scoring system for impending fracture has demonstrated good specificity for femoral fractures (Goodheart, Cleary, Damron, & Mann, 2015) and acceptable sensitivity for humeral fractures (Evans, Bottros, Grant, Chen, & Damron, 2008). Nonoperative interventions include radiation therapy, pain management, chemotherapy, endocrine therapy, bisphosphonates, external orthoses, and weight-bearing restrictions.

Physical activity for cancer survivors with skeletal metastases should focus on maintaining functional mobility and improving balance to reduce the risk of falls. Home safety evaluations can provide recommendations on fall risk reduction within the survivor's environment. Body mechanics training should address safe lifting techniques and the use of adaptive equipment for activities of daily living. Survivors should be provided appropriate assistive devices, gait training, and alternative means of mobility in instances of imposed weight-bearing restrictions. Medical necessity should be determined for wheelchairs and motorized mobility devices for survivors unable to self-propel.

Skeletal-Related Events

Skeletal-related events (SREs)—defined as pathologic fracture, spinal cord compression, the need for surgery or radiation therapy to the skeleton, or hypercalcemia—can be unfortunate sequelae of cancer and cancer treatment for many survivors. SREs associated with bone metastases can include pain, pathologic fracture, hypercalcemia, and neurologic deficits. Cancer survivors with skeletal metastases are at significant risk for SREs. Greater than 50% of breast cancer survivors with metastasis isolated to the skeleton experience SREs (Domchek, Younger, Finkelstein, & Seiden, 2000). A systematic review and meta-analysis by Wang et al. (2015) highlighted data from the untreated arms of several clinical trials, which indicated a two-year cumulative incidence of SREs as most prevalent in patients with skeletal metastasis with primary breast cancer (68%), prostate cancer (49%), and non-small cell lung cancer and other solid tumors (21-month cumulative incidence of 48%) (Lipton et al., 2000; Rosen et al., 2004; Saad, McKiernan, & Eastham, 2006).

Central Nervous System Metastases

According to the American Brain Tumor Association (ABTA, 2016), an estimated 100,000–170,000 central nervous system (CNS) metastases occur annually in the United States. Metastatic CNS lesions are the most common brain tumors in adults, occurring in an estimated 10%–30% of all cancer survivors; 80% of brain metastases occur in the cerebral hemispheres, 15% in the cerebellum, and 5% in the brain stem (Brastianos, Cahill, & Brastianos, 2015; Nabors et al., 2014). They arise most frequently as multiple lesions (ABTA, 2016).

Rehabilitation approaches with CNS metastases are intended to address and support cancer survivors' impairments. The visual, vestibular, motor, and sensory deficits, alone or in combination, can produce profound balance deficits. This can require interventions to reduce the risk of falls and improve patient safety. Significant motor deficits should be assessed for appropriate bracing or assistive devices for gait training.

Physical activity for individuals with CNS metastases must be tailored to their disease and clinical presentation. In the presence of balance deficits, caution should be taken for safety during positional changes. Using positions, including seated, supine, and a semireclined position (if indicated due to intracranial pressure), can offer improved safety during physical activity and exercise and reduce fall risk.

Pulmonary Metastases

According to Langley and Fidler (2011), the lung is the second most common site for distant metastasis. Individuals with pulmonary metastasis can present with respiratory symptoms more debilitating than the symptoms resulting from their primary cancer.

Prior to recommending physical activity to cancer survivors with pulmonary metastases, oncology nurses should perform a thorough review of the survivors' diagnostic imaging to assess the extent and location of the lesions. Close attention should be paid to metastases in the upper lobes because of the proximity to the cardiac circulation, as well as lesions in the mediastinal region, which may compromise the bronchi and the heart. Prior to initiation of physical activity, vitals monitoring at rest and with activity should include blood pressure, respiratory rate, oxygen saturation levels, and heart rate. During initial attempts at physical activity, cancer survivors with inoperable primary lung carcinoma or metastatic pulmonary lesions should be monitored for their current fatigue level (see Chapter 8), activity tolerance, and level of dyspnea. For survivors on supplemental oxygen, an order should be obtained to increase the liters, should their oxygen saturation level drop below 90% on pulse oximetry during physical activity. Patient education on diaphragmatic and pursed-lip breathing techniques incorporated into physical activity may assist survivors in controlling their respiratory rate. Performing exercises while sitting can help to conserve energy in survivors who easily become dyspneic while standing or walking. Instructing cancer survivors to lean forward in the sitting position while resting their hands on their knees can help to reduce symptoms of breathlessness for some. Adjusting physical activity intensity based on rating of perceived exertion, such as ratings on the Borg scale (see Chapter 7), can improve exercise tolerance and accuracy of an exercise prescription.

Widespread Metastases

In survivors with evidence of disseminated metastatic disease, oncology nurses should be aware of the location and extent of all metastases. These individuals often present with a multitude of symptoms. Each additional lesion can present with additional complications, and metastasis in one area can compound the symptoms resulting from metastasis elsewhere. The cumulative effects of disease-related symptoms, multiple medications, and organ system failures can cause varying presentations over time and from day to day. Cancer survivors should be educated on maximizing their abilities on days that permit, while allowing for rest on days when they are more symptomatic. These individuals require close monitoring for new symptom presentation or existing symptom progression; therefore, the skill of an oncology-trained physical therapist is recommended to prescribe physical activity in these complex cases.

For survivors with a limited performance status, a homecare therapist can provide several options. Survivors with limited ambulatory endurance can be prescribed an interval walking program of short distances on level surfaces with or without an assistive device multiple times per day. Individuals with limited ambulatory tolerance can be prescribed standing exercises performed while holding onto a secure surface for safety in order to maintain functional lower extremity muscle strength. Survivors spending the majority of time either in a chair or bed should be prescribed exercises in sitting or supine positions for both range of motion and isometric strengthening. With multiple options, survivors still can maintain some degree of physical activity regardless of their capabilities on any given day. Emphasizing and encouraging cancer survivors' abilities in their current state, while keeping safety in mind, will empower to the individual and yield the best outcomes. Figure 13-3 suggests steps in exercise progression for individuals with advanced cancer. Table 13-2 summarizes common metastatic sites, symptoms, and evidence on physical activity.

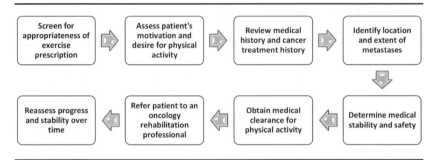

Figure 13-3. Steps in Exercise Prescription for Individuals With Advanced Cancer

Application to Oncology Nursing Practice

Oncology Nursing Assessment

1. Review cancer survivors' health history to determine if they have been diagnosed with metastatic disease.
2. Obtain your oncology center's current guidelines for caring for survivors with metastatic disease. Compare your center's practice with the evidence presented in this chapter.
3. Determine if a referral for additional oncologic services is needed, such as physical and occupational therapy, nutrition services, or hospice services.

Self-Report and Physical Activity Assessment

1. Assess current physical activity patterns using measures such as those described in Chapter 4.
2. Use the physical activity and exercise measures endorsed by your oncology center to measure activity. Assessing cancer survivors' current physical activ-

Table 13-2. Summary of Common Metastatic Sites, Symptoms, and Evidence on Physical Activity

Metastatic Site	Most Common Sites of Origin	Common Symptoms	Evidence to Support Physical Activity
Skeletal	Malignancies of the breast (73%), prostate (68%), and lung (36%) (Coleman, 2006) Langley and Fidler (2011) reported incidence rates of bone metastases in breast cancers (65%–75%), prostate cancers (68%), and lung and kidney cancers (40%).	Reduction in quality of life and often early mortality (Agarwal & Nayak, 2015) Pain, pathologic fracture, spinal lesions, and/ or risk of spinal cord compression (Tordiglione et al., 1999)	Guided isometric resistance training of the paravertebral muscles can improve functional capacity and reduce fatigue, thereby enhancing quality of life over a six-month period in patients with stable spinal metastases (Rief et al., 2014).
Central nervous system	Melanoma and lung, breast, colon, and kidney cancers commonly spread to the brain (American Brain Tumor Association [ABTA], 2015).	Headache; seizures; nausea and vomiting; visual, vestibular, and hearing changes; altered speech; fatigue; lethargy; memory and communication deficits; motor deficits, resulting in hyper- or hypotonicity, weakness, and/or incoordination; sensory and/or proprioception deficits; and psychosocial and emotional issues (ABTA, 2015)	Bartolo et al. (2012) assessed the functional outcomes of 75 patients who had undergone neurosurgery for primary brain tumors and 75 patients affected by stroke in a case-control study. They found that all outcome measures (Functional Independence Measure, Sitting Balance score, Standing Balance score, Hauser Index, and Massachusetts General Hospital Functional Ambulation Classification) were indicative of substantial improvements for neuro-oncology patients and for patients who experienced a stroke ($p = 0.000$). These findings may have implications for patients with metastatic brain lesions as well, but one should extrapolate the results with caution.

(Continued on next page)

Table 13-2. Summary of Common Metastatic Sites, Symptoms, and Evidence on Physical Activity *(Continued)*

Metastatic Site	Most Common Sites of Origin	Common Symptoms	Evidence to Support Physical Activity
Liver	Cutaneous melanoma; lung, colon, and breast cancer; and neuroendocrine tumors (Langley & Fidler, 2011)	Anorexia, jaundice, weight loss, nausea, confusion, pain (often in the right upper abdomen), and ascites (U.S. National Library of Medicine, 2014a)	Ascites may limit patient comfort and trunk flexibility during physical activity; therefore, prescribing exercises that limit repetitive trunk flexion or hip flexion greater than 90° may improve exercise tolerance. For patients receiving paracentesis on a routine basis for palliation, physical activity may be more easily tolerated in the days following the procedure.
Pulmonary	Primary breast, bladder, colon, kidney, head and neck, and skin cancer (melanoma) have an affinity to metastasize to the lung.	Shortness of breath, cough, weight loss, chest pain, bloody sputum, and weakness (U.S. National Library of Medicine, 2014b)	Yates et al. (2013) reviewed supportive and palliative care for patients with lung cancer experiencing dyspnea and highlighted nonpharmacologic interventions to improve breathing efficiency. This included pursed-lip breathing, diaphragmatic breathing, "blow-as-you-go," and positioning and pacing techniques. Bausewein et al. (2008) completed a systematic review of 47 studies with 2,532 participants who experienced breathlessness. The authors determined that breathing training, walking aids, neuromuscular electrical stimulation, and chest wall vibration appeared to be effective nonpharmacologic interventions for relieving breathlessness in advanced stages of disease.

ities assists the oncology nurse in understanding the level of physical activity in which survivors are currently engaged.

3. Evaluate the relationship between cancer survivors' physical activity and degree of metastatic disease. Assess the frequency, intensity, time, and type of activities. Are the types of activities too strenuous for the cancer survivor? Is the survivor in too much pain or having other health issues that prevent participation in activities of daily living?

4. Determine if a consultation to a physical or occupational therapist is indicated if functional mobility impairments are noted.

Oncology Nursing Recommendations for Physical Activity for Metastatic Disease

1. Use any of the interviewing techniques discussed in Chapter 5 to determine survivors' readiness to incorporate physical activity and exercise into their lifestyle.

2. Teach survivors about the potential benefits of staying physically active at levels that are best for them.

3. Use the evidence presented in this chapter to create a patient education fact sheet and use the education materials provided by your oncology center. Assure survivors that an individualized physical activity program can benefit them.

4. Collaborate with survivors to select physical activities and exercises they enjoy and are able to perform regularly and safely. Use checklists offered by your oncology center or the lists provided in Chapters 1 and 4.

5. Encourage cancer survivors to report moderate to severe symptoms after starting physical activity in order to discuss ways to reduce these symptoms.

6. Select a method for tracking physical activity, if desired. Ask survivors to bring the tracking program with them on their next visit.

Oncology Nursing Evaluation of Health Outcomes

1. Evaluate cancer survivors' ability to engage in the recommended physical activities. Note any improvements in or worsening of their health status.

2. Revise the physical activity plan as needed. Adjust the frequency, intensity, time, and type of activities to meet survivors' needs.

3. Follow up with referrals for physical or occupational therapy, nutrition services, and hospice as required by your oncology center.

Summary

It is imperative that palliative rehabilitation measures focus on maintaining the dignity and preservation of cancer survivors. Survivors with metastatic disease may experience a multitude of symptoms, some of which may be alleviated by physical activity. Physical activity has become an available and accepted option for long-term cancer survivors in regard to managing symptoms and providing patients with a sense of control. It is important to encourage cancer survivors to participate in physical activity and exercise as they are able in order to provide empowerment to individuals and yield positive outcomes.

Case Study

(Continued from Chapter 12)

Patient presentation: New-onset headaches and balance issues. Magnetic resonance imaging scan of the brain revealed multiple metastases to the cerebellum.

Plan of care: Radiation therapy to whole brain; temozolomide, dexamethasone, and phenytoin

12 months later

Patient presentation: New onset of low back pain. A bone scan reveals osteolytic bone metastases to the fourth lumbar vertebrae (L4) and mixed osteoblastic/osteolytic bone metastases to right (R) and left (L) pelvis (mid-R ilium to superior aspect of R acetabulum) (8 cm), L iliac crest (2–4 cm), R proximal femur (2.5 cm), and L eighth rib.

Plan of care: D.J. is made non–weight-bearing (NWB) on R lower extremity immediately after her computed tomography simulation. Orthopedic consultation with a hip surgeon followed, and prophylactic surgery is considered unnecessary. D.J. is considered at a high risk for pathologic fracture. Radiation therapy to L4. Radiation therapy to L pelvis and R femur (10 fractions each). Radiation therapy to rib (five fractions). Zoledronic acid also is initiated.

What would be best to help support D.J.?
Services provided include the following:
- Further counseling for D.J. and her husband for adjustment to progressive illness
- Palliative care consultation with admission to the advanced illness program
- Homecare consultation for both physical therapy and occupational therapy
- Adaptive equipment for home secured through patient support fund to improve independence with activities of daily living (e.g., tub seat, elevated toilet seat)
- Mobility equipment, including a low-profile wheelchair, which will allow for self-propulsion, and spring-loaded ergonomic axillary crutches (for transition from NWB in wheelchair, to NWB on crutches, to partial weight-bearing, to weight-bearing as tolerated, to full weight-bearing)
- Massage therapy continued on an inpatient and outpatient basis
- Spiritual care consultation and counseling provided in radiation therapy center

---

Follow-Up
After completing radiation therapy and returning to full weight-bearing, D.J. participates in a randomized exercise study for patients with stage IV cancer and was randomized to the cardiovascular group. She completes 20/20 (100%) prescribed sessions, with an average of 47.5 minutes of aerobic exercise per session (water walking

in the pool and an upper body ergometer). D.J. returns to her independent gym membership with appropriate safety modifications, precautions, and risk education. Topotecan is initiated for chemotherapy.

Patient presentation: Severe lethargy, confusion, and difficulty with transferring from sitting to standing while in the waiting room. Neutropenic fever with septic shock was diagnosed, and D.J. was admitted to the intensive care unit for a three-night stay for IV antibiotics.
- D.J. recovered from infection and was discharged to home with hospice support.
- Hospice was able to provide pain control with a fentanyl transdermal system and oxycodone.
- D.J. and her husband were able to enjoy the birth of a grandchild that spring.
- D.J. presented with refractory cachexia but maintained good skin integrity and functional mobility.
- D.J. was able to maintain her mobility safely and never had a fall at home.
- She died peacefully at home surrounded by family at age 53.
- Hospice provided bereavement services to her family to help them cope with their loss.

An initial diagnosis of stage IV cancer is never easy to process or accept. This patient experienced metastasis in three different organ systems and had to endure many different treatment plans during the course of her progressive illness. Her case required special consideration. Despite all the challenges she faced due to her terminal illness, including a poor prognosis and a cancer-related emergency, she remained in control of her supportive care and symptom management. She took full advantage of the interprofessional services available to her and her family and embraced the care the team was able to provide. This chapter is dedicated to her memory and to all the patients who have walked the path with her.

References

Agarwal, M.G., & Nayak, P. (2015). Management of skeletal metastases: An orthopaedic surgeon's guide. *Indian Journal of Orthopaedics, 49,* 83–100. doi:10.4103/0019-5413.143915

American Brain Tumor Association. (2015). Brain tumor symptoms. Retrieved from http://www.abta.org/brain-tumor-information/symptoms

American Brain Tumor Association. (2016). Metastatic brain tumors. Retrieved from http://www.abta.org/secure/metastatic-brain-tumor.pdf

Bartolo, M., Zucchella, C., Pace, A., Lanzetta, G., Vecchione, C., Bartolo, M., ... Pierelli, F. (2012). Early rehabilitation after surgery improves functional outcome in inpatients with brain tumours. *Journal of Neuro-Oncology, 107,* 537–544. doi:10.1007/s11060-011-0772-5

Bausewein, C., Booth, S., Gysels, M., & Higginson, I.J. (2008). Non-pharmacological interventions for breathlessness in advanced stages of malignant and non-malignant diseases. *Cochrane Database of Systematic Reviews, 2008*(2). doi:10.1002/14651858.CD005623.pub2

Beaton, R., Pagdin-Friesen, W., Robertson, C., Vigar, C., Watson, H., & Harris, S.R. (2009). Effects of exercise intervention on persons with metastatic cancer: A systematic review. *Physiotherapy Canada, 61,* 141–153. doi:10.3138/physio.61.3.141

Brant, J.M., & Wickham, R. (Eds.). (2013). *Statement on the scope and standards of oncology nursing practice: Generalist and advanced practice.* Pittsburgh, PA: Oncology Nursing Society.

Brastianos, H.C., Cahill, D.P., & Brastianos, P.K. (2015). Systemic therapy of brain metastases. *Current Neurology and Neuroscience Reports, 15,* 518. doi:10.1007/s11910-014-0518-9

Cheville, A.L., Kollasch, J., Vandenberg, J., Shen, T., Grothey, A., Gamble, G., & Basford, J.R. (2013). A home-based exercise program to improve function, fatigue, and sleep quality in patients with stage IV lung and colorectal cancer: A randomized controlled trial. *Journal of Pain and Symptom Management, 45,* 811–821. doi:10.1016/j.jpainsymman.2012.05.006

Cheville, A.L., Troxel, A.B., Basford, J.R., & Kornblith, A.B. (2008). Prevalence and treatment patterns of physical impairments in patients with metastatic breast cancer. *Journal of Clinical Oncology, 26,* 2621–2629. doi:10.1200/JCO.2007.12.3075

Chow, E., Harris, K., Fan, G., Tsao, M., & Sze, W.M. (2007). Palliative radiotherapy trials for bone metastases: A systematic review. *Journal of Clinical Oncology, 25,* 1423–1436. doi:10.1200/JCO.2006.09.5281

Coleman, R.E. (2006). Clinical features of metastatic bone disease and risk of skeletal morbidity. *Clinical Cancer Research, 12,* 6243s. doi:10.1158/1078-0432.CCR-06-0931

Dietz, J. (1981). *Rehabilitation oncology.* New York, NY: John Wiley and Sons.

Domchek, S.M., Younger, J., Finkelstein, D.M., & Seiden, M.V. (2000). Predictors of skeletal complications in patients with metastatic breast carcinoma. *Cancer, 89,* 363–368.

Evans, A.R., Bottros, J., Grant, W., Chen, B.Y., & Damron, T.A. (2008). Mirels' rating for humerus lesions is both reproducible and valid. *Clinical Orthopaedics and Related Research, 466,* 1279–1284. doi:10.1007/s11999-008-0200-0

Goodheart, J.R., Cleary, R.J., Damron, T.A., & Mann, K.A. (2015). Simulating activities of daily living with finite element analysis improves fracture prediction for patients with metastatic femoral lesions. *Journal of Orthopaedic Research, 33,* 1226–1234. doi:10.1002/jor.22887

Krishna, L.K.R., Yong, C.Y.L., & Koh, S.M.C. (2014). The role of palliative rehabilitation in the preservation of personhood at the end of life. *BMJ Case Reports, 2014.* doi:10.1136/bcr-2014-204780

Langley, R.R., & Fidler, I.J. (2011). The seed and soil hypothesis revisited—The role of tumor-stroma interactions in metastasis to different organs. *International Journal of Cancer, 128,* 2527–2535. doi:10.1002/ijc.26031

Lipton, A., Theriault, R.L., Hortobagyi, G.N., Simeone, J., Knight, R.D., Mellars, K., ... Seaman, J.J. (2000). Pamidronate prevents skeletal complications and is effective palliative treatment in women with breast carcinoma and osteolytic bone metastases: Long-term follow-up of two randomized, placebo-controlled trials. *Cancer, 88,* 1082–1090.

Litterini, A.J., & Fieler, V. (2008). The change in fatigue, strength, and quality of life following a physical therapist prescribed exercise program for cancer survivors. *Rehabilitation Oncology, 26,* 11–17.

Litterini, A.J., Fieler, V.K., Cavanaugh, J.T., & Lee, J.Q. (2013). Differential effects of cardiovascular and resistance exercise on functional mobility in individuals with advanced cancer: A randomized trial. *Archives of Physical Medicine and Rehabilitation, 94,* 2329–2335. doi:10.1016/j.apmr.2013.06.008

Lowe, S.S., Watanabe, S.M., Baracos, V.E., & Courneya, K.S. (2010). Physical activity interests and preferences in palliative cancer patients. *Supportive Care in Cancer, 18,* 1469–1475. doi:10.1007/s00520-009-0770-8

Lutz, S., Berk, L., Chang, E., Chow, E., Hahn, C., Hoskin, P., ... Hartsell, W. (2011). Palliative radiotherapy for bone metastases: An ASTRO evidence-based guideline. *International Journal of Radiation Oncology, Biology, Physics, 79,* 965–976. doi:10.1016/j.ijrobp.2010.11.026

Mirels, H. (2003). Metastatic disease in long bones. A proposed scoring system for diagnosing impending pathologic fractures. 1989. *Clinical Orthopaedics and Related Research, 415*(Suppl.), S4–S13.

Mishra, S.I., Scherer, R.W., Geigle, P.M., Berlanstein, D.R., Topaloglu, O., Gotay, C.C., & Snyder, C. (2012). Exercise interventions on health-related quality of life for cancer survivors. *Cochrane Database of Systematic Reviews, 2012*(8). doi:10.1002/14651858.CD007566.pub2

Nabors, L.B., Portnow, J., Ammirati, M., Brem, H., Brown, P., Butowski, N., ... Ho, M. (2014). Central nervous system cancers, version 2.2014. Featured updates to the NCCN Guidelines. *Journal of the National Comprehensive Cancer Network, 12,* 1517–1523.

National Comprehensive Cancer Network. (2016). *NCCN Clinical Practice Guidelines in Oncology (NCCN Guidelines®): Cancer-related fatigue* [v.1.2016]. Retrieved from http://www.nccn.org/professionals/physician_gls/PDF/fatigue.pdf

Norden, A.D., Wen, P.Y., & Kesari, S. (2005). Brain metastases. *Current Opinion in Neurology, 18,* 654–661.

Payne, C., Larkin, P.J., McIlfatrick, S., Dunwoody, L., & Gracey, J.H. (2013). Exercise and nutrition interventions in advanced lung cancer: A systematic review. *Current Oncology, 20,* E321–E337. doi:10.3747/co.20.1431

Quist, M., Rørth, M., Langer, S., Jones, L.W., Laursen, J.H., Pappot, H., … Adamsen, L. (2012). Safety and feasibility of a combined exercise intervention for inoperable lung cancer patients undergoing chemotherapy: A pilot study. *Lung Cancer, 75,* 203–208.

Rief, H., Akbar, M., Keller, M., Omlor, G., Welzel, T., Bruckner, T., … Debus, J. (2014). Quality of life and fatigue of patients with spinal bone metastases under combined treatment with resistance training and radiation therapy—A randomized pilot trial. *Radiation Oncology, 9,* 151. doi:10.1186/1748-717X-9-151

Rock, C.L., Doyle, C., Demark-Wahnefried, W., Meyerhardt, J., Courneya, K.S., Schwartz, A.L., … Gansler, T. (2012). Nutrition and physical activity guidelines for cancer survivors. *CA: A Cancer Journal for Clinicians, 62,* 243–274. doi:10.3322/caac.21142

Rosen, L.S., Gordon, D., Tchekmedyian, N.S., Yanagihara, R., Hirsh, V., Krzakowski, M., … Seaman, J. (2004). Long-term efficacy and safety of zoledronic acid in the treatment of skeletal metastases in patients with nonsmall cell lung carcinoma and other solid tumors. *Cancer, 100,* 2613–2621. doi:10.1002/cncr.20308

Ruijs, C.D., Kerkhof, A.J., van der Wal, G., & Onwuteaka-Philipsen, B.D. (2013). Symptoms, unbearability and the nature of suffering in terminal cancer patients dying at home: A prospective primary care study. *BMC Family Practice, 14,* 201. doi:10.1186/1471-2296-14-201

Saad, F., McKiernan, J., & Eastham, J. (2006). Rationale for zoledronic acid therapy in men with hormone-sensitive prostate cancer with or without bone metastasis. *Urologic Oncology, 24,* 4–12. doi:10.1016/j.urolonc.2005.06.020

Studenski, S., Perera, S., Patel, K., Rosano, C., Faulkner, K., Inzitari, M., … Guralnik, J. (2011). Gait speed and survival in older adults. *JAMA, 305,* 50–58. doi:10.1001/jama.2010.1923

Temel, J., Greer, J., Goldberg, S., Vogel, P.D., Sullivan, M., Lynch, T.J., … Smith, M.R. (2009). A structured exercise program for patients with advanced non-small cell lung cancer. *Journal of Thoracic Oncology, 4,* 595–601. doi:10.1097/JTO.0b013e31819d18e5

Tordiglione, M., Luraghi, R., & Antognoni, P. (1999). Role of palliative and symptomatic radiotherapy in bone metastasis. *La Radiologia Medica, 97,* 372–377.

U.S. National Library of Medicine. (2014a). Liver metastases. Retrieved from http://www.nlm.nih.gov/medlineplus/ency/article/000277.htm

U.S. National Library of Medicine. (2014b). Lung metastases. Retrieved from http://www.nlm.nih.gov/medlineplus/ency/article/000097.htm

Wang, Z., Qiao, D., Lu, Y., Curtis, D., Wen, X., Yao, Y., & Zhao, H. (2015). Systematic literature review and network meta-analysis comparing bone-targeted agents for the prevention of skeletal-related events in cancer patients with bone metastasis. *Oncologist, 20,* 440–449. doi:10.1634/theoncologist.2014-0328

Yates, P., Schofield, P., Zhao, I., & Currow, D. (2013). Supportive and palliative care for lung cancer patients. *Journal of Thoracic Disease, 5*(Suppl. 5), S623–S628.

CHAPTER 14

Physical Activity and Cancer Survival: Future Directions

Kerry S. Courneya, PhD, Andria R. Morielli, MSc, and Linda Trinh, PhD

Introduction

Overwhelming research and evidence-based guidelines support the benefits of physical activity and exercise for cancer survivors. For over 25 years, the field of exercise oncology has matured, and ongoing interdisciplinary research continues to add progress to this emerging field (Jones & Alfano, 2013). Oncology nurses can integrate the current research and guidelines into their nursing practice to improve cancer survivors' experience with physical activity and exercise. This chapter describes ongoing and future research that will advance the science of physical activity and exercise in cancer survivorship. This chapter's content is supported in the Oncology Nursing Society's *Statement on the Scope and Standards of Oncology Nursing Practice: Generalist and Advanced Practice* (Brant & Wickham, 2013) (see Figure 14-1).

Ongoing Research: Physical Activity and Breast Cancer Outcomes

Although the data on exercise and breast cancer outcomes are promising (see Chapter 2), the studies have been limited by self-reported measures and secondary analyses of studies that were not originally designed to answer this question. Clinical studies currently underway are described in this chapter.

Alberta Moving Beyond Breast Cancer Cohort Study

Alberta Moving Beyond Breast Cancer (AMBER) is designed specifically to focus on the role of physical activity and health-related fitness in breast cancer survivors (Courneya et al., 2012). AMBER is enrolling 1,500 newly diagnosed, stage I (≥ stage T1c) to stage IIIc breast cancer survivors within a few months of diagnosis. Assessments will be made at baseline and at one, three, and five years with follow-up consisting of objective (i.e., accelerometers) and self-reported measurements of physical activity, sedentary behavior, and health-

---

Standard VIII. Education
- Identify personal knowledge deficits and pursue educational opportunities (e.g., academic education, simulated and actual clinical skills training, accredited continuing education, self-paced learning via oncology nursing publications) to expand clinical knowledge and enhance role performance.
- Seek information from non-oncology sources to expand knowledge that may potentially affect the care of patients with cancer, for example, long-term organ-effect management in survivors, general genetics principles, and psychosocial care issues. The nurse evaluates application of this scientific and clinical knowledge to cancer care.
- Seek innovative oncology experiences and educational opportunities in all aspects of cancer care to maintain knowledge, attitudes, skills, abilities, clinical judgment, and behaviors in clinical practice and role performance.

Standard IX. Evidence-Based Practice and Research
- Regularly access nationally recognized clinical practice guidelines (e.g., Oncology Nursing Society position statements and Putting Evidence Into Practice resources; American Society of Clinical Oncology and National Comprehensive Cancer Network clinical practice guidelines) to support evidence-based patient care and teaching.
- Base clinical decision making and delivery of individualized patient care on best current evidence, patient values and preferences, and resource availability.
- Facilitate integration of new evidence into standards of practice, development or modification of policies, practice guidelines, education, and clinical management strategies.

Standard XII. Leadership
- Anticipate oncology and healthcare trends with changes such as innovative practice settings and models of care delivery, increased focus on older adult patients and cancer survivors, and technological advances that affect care.

Figure 14-1. Standards Applicable to Future Research in Physical Activity and Cancer Survivors

---

Note. From *Statement on the Scope and Standards of Oncology Nursing Practice: Generalist and Advanced Practice,* by J.M. Brant and R. Wickham (Eds.), 2013, Pittsburgh, PA: Oncology Nursing Society. Copyright 2013 by Oncology Nursing Society. Adapted with permission.

related fitness. Blood samples also will be taken at this time to assess important biomarkers that potentially are associated with physical activity and breast cancer outcomes. AMBER will provide valuable information on the type, volume, intensity, and timing of physical activity that is optimal for improving breast cancer outcomes and survivorship.

Supervised Trial of Aerobic Versus Resistance Training

Supervised Trial of Aerobic Versus Resistance Training (START) provided the first randomized phase II data on the effects of exercise on breast cancer outcomes (Courneya, Segal, et al., 2014). START was a multicenter trial that randomized 242 patients with breast cancer who were starting adjuvant chemotherapy to either usual care (n = 82) or supervised aerobic (n = 78) or resistance (n = 82) exercise for the duration of their chemotherapy. The two exercise arms were combined for analysis (n = 160), and selected subgroups were explored. After a median follow-up of 89 months, disease-free survival of eight years was 82.7% for the exercise groups compared to 75.6% for the usual care group (hazard ratio [HR] = 0.68; 95% confidence interval [0.37–1.24]; log-rank p = 0.21). Stronger effects were observed for overall survival, distant disease-free survival, and recurrence-free interval. Subgroup analyses suggested stronger effects for women who were overweight or obese, had stage II or III cancer, had estrogen receptor–positive or HER2-positive tumors, received taxane-based chemotherapies, and had received at least 85% of their intended chemotherapy dose intensity. This exploratory follow-up of START provided the first randomized data to suggest that adding exercise to standard chemotherapy for breast cancer may improve outcomes.

Influence of Exercise on Neurocognitive Function in Breast Cancer

In healthy older adults, exercise interventions have been demonstrated to improve memory, executive function, and psychomotor efficiency (Erickson, Gildengers, & Butters, 2013), the very cognitive domains that decline with endocrine therapy in breast cancer (Bender et al., 2015). A new study is being designed to determine whether a six-month, moderate-intensity aerobic exercise intervention improves cognitive function and brain function. The study will use neuroimaging techniques in postmenopausal women with early-stage breast cancer who receive aromatase inhibitor therapy (Bender, Erickson, Marsland, & Sereika, 2016). This study is a clinical trial in which participants are randomized to the aerobic exercise intervention or usual care group before they begin aromatase inhibitor therapy. The study also will determine whether aerobic exercise reduces levels of proinflammatory biomarkers and symptoms associated with breast cancer and breast cancer therapy (e.g., fatigue, sleep problems, depression, anxiety) (Bender et al., 2016).

Ongoing Research: Physical Activity and Colorectal Cancer Outcomes

Similar to the studies of physical activity in breast cancer survivors, all of the studies to date that have examined exercise and colorectal cancer outcomes have been observational cohort studies. Consequently, it is possible that the associations between physical activity and cancer outcomes are due to some other factors (e.g., active cancer survivors are in better health, have less aggressive disease, are fitter, are more likely to take care of themselves). To address this issue, randomized controlled trials are needed. One such study that is ongoing is the Colon Health and Life-Long Exercise Change (CHALLENGE) Trial (Courneya et al., 2008; Courneya, Vardy, et al., 2014).

CHALLENGE is designed to determine the effects of a structured physical activity intervention on disease outcomes in high-risk stage II and III colon cancer survivors who have completed chemotherapy within the past two to six months (Courneya et al., 2008; Courneya, Vardy, et al., 2014). The study will recruit 962 colon cancer survivors and randomly assign them to a structured physical activity intervention or general health education materials.

The physical activity intervention will consist of behavioral counseling and some supervised exercise sessions over a three-year period. CHALLENGE will provide important data on the causal effects of physical activity on disease recurrence and survival in colorectal cancer survivors that can be used to develop effective physical activity programs for this population.

Ongoing Research: Physical Activity and Prostate Cancer Outcomes

Provocative evidence supports the beneficial role of physical activity on prostate cancer survivorship. Evaluating exercise as a low-toxicity adjuvant intervention that can be combined with standard therapy to improve outcomes in men with prostate cancer could reduce the clinical and public health burden of the disease. Exercise may affect prostate cancer survival via inflammation, hormonal changes, and energy metabolism pathways.

A prospective randomized controlled clinical trial, the INTense Exercise foR surVivAL Among Men With Metastatic Castrate-Resistant Prostate Cancer (INTERVAL) trial, was designed to compare overall survival among men with metastatic castrate-resistant prostate cancer (MCRPC). Participants are randomly assigned to psychosocial support with or without high-intensity aerobic and resistance training for 24 months. Secondary outcomes include time to progression; occurrence of skeletal-related events; progression of pain; and degree of pain, opiate use, and physical and emotional quality of life. Study measures will determine if inflammation, dysregulation of insulin and energy metabolism, and androgen biomarkers are associated with overall survival and if they mediate the primary association between exercise and overall survival.

INTERVAL will establish a biobank for future biomarker discovery or validation. This multisite global trial will include patients with MCRPC who are treatment naïve or on abiraterone acetate or enzalutamide without evidence of progression at enrollment. Patients will be randomized (1:1) to psychosocial support with or without high-intensity aerobic and resistance training (Saad et al., 2016).

The first 12 months of training will include a structured period of tapered supervised exercise, with increasing self-managed exercise and behavioral support with text messages to support self-management for an additional 12 months. Exercise prescriptions will be tailored to participants' fitness and cancer/treatment morbidities.

Assuming a median overall survival rate of 33.5 months in the controls, the sample size to detect an HR of 0.78 with 80% power at significance level of 0.05 is 824; assuming missing data on overall survival for 5%, the goal is to enroll 866 men (Saad et al., 2016). This is the first prospective randomized trial to examine exercise and survival in men with prostate cancer and is designed to elucidate the mechanisms by which exercise delays cancer progression.

Application to Oncology Nursing Practice

1. Learn more about ongoing clinical trials that measure the effect of physical activity and exercise in cancer survivors by visiting http://clinicaltrials .gov. This website provides a list of government-funded research that is either ongoing, closed, or not yet open for recruitment. Read the synopses for studies that are of interest to you. Discuss these trials with your oncology team to determine if they are appropriate for your center's population.

2. Visit reputable websites related to oncology nursing, oncology, and exercise science (see Chapter 15) to learn more about research trials and published research.

3. Become involved in physical activity and exercise research with cancer survivors at your oncology center. Read evidence-based articles and share insights with your oncology team. Participate in a journal club, blog, or other dissemination method to share information about this topic.

4. Find a mentor who focuses on physical activity and exercise in cancer survivors. Participate with your mentor in writing abstracts, applying for grants, and preparing manuscripts and presentations. Decide if this is a specialty area that you would like to pursue.

5. Become involved in professional organizations, such as the Oncology Nursing Society (www.ons.org), that promote physical activity and exercise in

cancer survivors and others. Contribute to your professional organization by participating in local, state, and national committees and events.

Summary

The relationship between physical activity and exercise and positive health outcomes in cancer survivors cannot be ignored. Research in the area of physical activity and cancer survivorship will continue to grow. Learning about ongoing research, applying research findings to practice, and becoming involved in professional organizations that support physical activity and cancer survivorship are within the realm of oncology nursing practice.

References

Bender, C.M., Erickson, K., Marsland, A., & Sereika, S.M. (2016). Influence of exercise on neurocognitive function in breast cancer. Unpublished raw data.

Bender, C.M., Merriman, J.D., Gentry, A.L., Ahrendt, G.M., Berga, S.L., Brufsky, A.M., ... Sereika, S.M. (2015). Patterns of change in cognitive function with anastrozole therapy. *Cancer, 121*, 2627–2636. doi:10.1002/cncr.29393

Brant, J.M., & Wickham, R. (Eds.). (2013). *Statement on the scope and standards of oncology nursing practice: Generalist and advanced practice.* Pittsburgh, PA: Oncology Nursing Society.

Courneya, K.S., Booth, C.M., Gill, S., O'Brien, P., Vardy, J., Friedenreich, C.M., ... Meyer, R.M. (2008). The Colon Health and Life-Long Exercise Change Trial: A randomized trial of the National Cancer Institute of Canada Clinical Trials Group. *Current Oncology, 15*, 271–278.

Courneya, K.S., Segal, R.J., McKenzie, D.C., Dong, H., Gelmon, K., Friedenreich, C.M., ... Mackey, J.R. (2014). Effects of exercise during adjuvant chemotherapy on breast cancer outcomes. *Medicine and Science in Sports and Exercise, 46*, 1744–1751. doi:10.1249/MSS.0000000000000297

Courneya, K.S., Vallance, J.K., Culos-Reed, S.N., McNeely, M.L., Bell, G.J., Mackey, J.R., ... Friedenreich, C.M. (2012). The Alberta Moving Beyond Breast Cancer (AMBER) cohort study: A prospective study of physical activity and health-related fitness in breast cancer survivors. *BMC Cancer, 12*, 525. doi:10.1186/1471-2407-12-525

Courneya, K.S., Vardy, J., Gill, S., Jonker, D., O'Brien, P., Friedenreich, C.M., ... Booth, C.M. (2014). Update on the Colon Health and Life-Long Exercise Change Trial: A phase III study of the impact of an exercise program on disease-free survival in colon cancer survivors. *Current Colorectal Cancer Reports, 10*, 321–328. doi:10.1007/s11888-014-0231-8

Erickson, K.I., Gildengers, A.G., & Butters, M.A. (2013). Physical activity and brain plasticity in late adulthood. *Dialogues in Clinical Neuroscience, 15*, 99–108.

Jones, L.W., & Alfano, C.M. (2013). Exercise-oncology research: Past, present, and future. *Acta Oncologica, 52*, 195–215. doi:10.3109/0284186X.2012.742564

Saad, F., Kenfield, S., Chan, J., Hart, N., Courneya, K., Catto, J., ... Newton, R. (2016). INTense Exercise foR surVivAL among men with metastatic castrate-resistant prostate cancer. Retrieved from http://www.trialdetails.com/detail/NCT02730338/INTense-Exercise-foR-surVivAL-Among -Men-With-Metastatic-Castrate-Resistant-Prostate-Cancer

CHAPTER 15

Support Groups and Resources

Betsy J. Becker, PT, DPT, CLT-LANA, Olivia Huffman, PT, DPT, Kara Tischer, PT, DPT, and Kelly McCormick, PT, DPT

Introduction

A strong support network is beneficial to cancer survivors and may serve as a buffer for the emotional issues associated with the diagnosis of cancer. As the health, social, and psychosocial needs of survivors change, their support needs also may vary. Support plays a vital role when addressing the psychosocial issues and quality of life for not only the individual diagnosed with cancer but also the family and caregiver (John, Kawachi, Lathan, & Ayanian, 2014).

Support comes in a variety of forms, such as support groups, time with family and friends, encouragement from healthcare providers, and resources from professional and lay organizations. Oncology nurses can refer cancer survivors to support groups and organizations geared toward physical activity in order to help survivors and families as they transition through the treatment process and beyond. This chapter outlines the various types of physical activity support groups and resources available to oncology nurses, cancer survivors, and cancer centers.

Support Groups

The support group format may be a traditional one with a formally trained facilitator, such as an oncology nurse, who leads the discussion and offers sup-

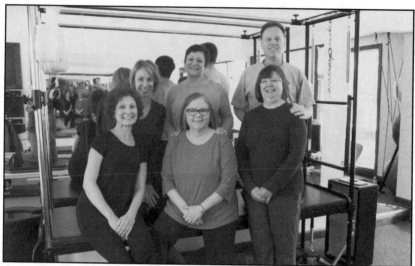

Supportive friends and family keep cancer survivors active and engaged in physical activity and exercise.

port and advice. An example of a more informal support group format would involve cancer survivors and caregivers sharing their experiences without the expertise of a trained professional. In a world where attaining information is easier than ever via the Internet, support may also be provided through online groups and social media.

Hoey, Ieropoli, White, and Jefford (2008) proposed that support groups are effective because they decrease isolation, encourage positive health behaviors, promote positive psychosocial states, and are a good source of information. The authors also noted that support groups serve as a buffer to the impact of emotions and stress by developing new coping responses and learned behaviors for survivors.

Models of support groups include face-to-face or group discussions, one-on-one or group phone calls, and online forums. In a systematic review of peer support groups, Hoey et al. (2008) reported that no one format is superior, but personal contact can help current cancer survivors in practical, social, and emotional ways. Like face-to-face groups, online support groups also have shown to improve quality of life, reduce distress, and positively affect psychosocial issues (Gorlick, Bantum, & Owen, 2014). The convenience and flexibility of online support groups may be appealing for individuals who have a busy schedule of medical appointments or work or family commitments or who prefer a more anonymous profile.

Support groups that meet in person have the benefit of very personal interactions in real time, which may be difficult to achieve online. This experience in the support group is important to consider when creating a support group or recommending one to cancer survivors. Connecting with others is an important component. Survivors could relate to similarities in diagnoses or treatment stage or make connections to those with similar demographics such as age (Gorlick et al., 2014). Cancer survivors who are not ready to share personal experiences can participate online by reading about others' experiences. This role is synonymous with attending a face-to-face group meeting but rarely speaking. In formally facilitated online support groups, users preferred interaction with the facilitator (Beck & Keyton, 2014; Gorlick et al., 2014).

Exercise-related support groups may be specific to cancer survivors, as exercises are designed for common impairments (e.g., decreased range of motion after surgery, fatigue related to cancer treatment). Individuals may already belong to existing exercise classes or groups, which may include the following:
• Group fitness classes: aerobic, strength/conditioning, stretching
• Exercise clubs: swim, crew, running, boxing

Examples of physical activity–specific groups in which cancer survivors participate may include the following:
• Walking groups: trail, neighborhood, mall
• Garden clubs
• Medical-based fitness centers
• Workplace wellness groups
• Sports-specific groups: golfing, fishing, billiards
• Recreation-specific groups: dance, chorus, board games
• Healing groups: meditation, yoga, mind–body fitness
• Online physical activity and exercise programs or applications in the home or workplace

Effectiveness of support groups is not universal and may not appeal to all people for a variety of reasons. A study of patients with lung cancer determined there are disparities in perceived unmet needs related to supportive care. Significant differences reported were related to race- and ethnicity-nativity and financial status. Unmet needs occur when there are differences in the services actually received by an individual compared to those deemed necessary to appropriately handle the issue (Carr & Wolk, 1976). Therefore, it is essential that oncology nurses be aware of cancer support and physical activity groups and resources available and advocate on the behalf of cancer survivors.

Resources

Cancer survivors can learn more about physical activity and exercise by visiting websites of professional and lay organizations that address physical activity and cancer survivorship. Oncology nurses can also benefit from learning about the processes used by these organizations to address physical activity and exercise in cancer survivors.

- Table 15-1 describes professional organizations that oncology nurses and cancer survivors may find helpful when learning more about the role of physical activity and exercise in cancer survivors. Oncology nurses can learn more about certifications and resources helpful in promoting physical activity and exercise in cancer survivors.
- Table 15-2 offers specific physical activity and exercise websites. These websites provide information about each exercise type. Based on this information, oncology nurses and cancer survivors can determine if the specific type of activity and exercise is appropriate and available in their geographic area.
- Table 15-3 lists professional organizations that provide outcome-specific measurements related to physical activity and exercise, as well as therapy. Oncology nurses may find these sites useful when measuring outcomes in patients and clients.
- Table 15-4 suggests lay organizations specific for cancer populations. Oncology nurses and survivors may find these sites helpful when exploring cancer-related treatment options and outcomes, as well as support services for specific types of cancers.

This is not an exhaustive list of resources. Oncology nurses can add to this list for use in their oncology center.

Table 15-1. Examples of Professional Organizations

Organization	Resources
Aerobics and Fitness Association of America www.afaa.com	Certification for group fitness and personal training
American Cancer Society www.cancer.org	Patient and caregiver information Infographics and research that may be helpful for patients
American College of Sports Medicine www.acsm.org	Exercise resources for professionals and the public Certifications for healthcare professionals (e.g., certified cancer exercise trainer, certified wellness coach) Programs for communities (e.g., Exercise is Medicine)
American Council on Exercise www.acefitness.org	Certification for fitness trainers Evidence-based health and fitness information for the public
American Occupational Therapy Association www.aota.org	Helpful tips on understanding what occupational therapists can bring to the team

(Continued on next page)

Table 15-1. Examples of Professional Organizations *(Continued)*

Organization	Resources
American Physical Therapy Association www.moveforwardpt.com/Default.aspx	Information for consumers about physical activity
American Therapeutic Recreation Association www.atra-online.com	Evidence, mentoring, and education to promote the profession of recreational therapy
Canadian Society for Exercise Physiology www.csep.ca	Resources to support the scientific study of exercise physiology, exercise biochemistry, fitness, and health
Lymphology Association of North America www.clt-lana.org	Certification for treating patients with lymphedema, continuing education offerings, and directory of lymphedema therapists
National Cancer Institute www.cancer.gov/about-cancer	Content for healthcare providers and patients
Oncology Rehab Partners—STAR (Survivorship Training and Rehab) Program www.starprogramoncologyrehab.com	Resources that can guide hospitals, cancer centers, and healthcare facilities when developing and implementing rehabilitation services for oncology (multidisciplinary)
SHAPE America www.shapeamerica.org	Support and assistance to professionals involved in physical education, recreation, fitness, sports and coaching, health education, and dance
Susan G. Komen http://ww5.komen.org	Research, treatment, screening, and education for patients with breast cancer

Application to Oncology Nursing Practice

1. Obtain a list of the cancer support groups utilized by your survivors. Determine the relevancy of the listed groups and which groups should be added or deleted.
2. Review the content of Table 15-1. Determine if you or your oncology center recommends any of the listed websites.
3. Ask cancer survivors about the activity and exercise groups in which they participate. Make a list of available groups to share with other cancer survivors.

Table 15-2. Examples of Professional Organizations for Cancer Survivors

Organization	Resources
American Cancer Society www.cancer.org	Research, patient services, early detection, treatment, and education
American Joint Committee on Cancer www.cancerstaging.org	Evidence-based system for cancer staging
American Physical Therapy Association (APTA) www.apta.org	Helpful tips on understanding what physical therapists can bring to the team
Association of Cancer Online Resources www.acor.org	Online support groups for different types of cancer
Cancer*Care* www.cancercare.org/professionals	Resources on counseling, continuing education, support groups, workshops, and publications
Cancer Index www.cancerindex.org	Index of websites such as research areas, oncology journals, treatment information, and organizations
Cancer Support Community www.cancersupportcommunity.org	Online support forum for family, friends, and caregivers
National Comprehensive Cancer Network® www.nccn.org	Care guidelines, resources, education, and links for support groups
National Institutes of Health ClinicalTrials.gov http://clinicaltrials.gov	List of all federally funded research (searchable by topic and location)
National Lymphedema Network www.lymphnet.org	Guidance and education for patients, healthcare professionals, and the general public about lymphedema risk, exercise, treatment, and diagnosis
Oncology Nursing Society www.ons.org	Evidence-based practice (including Putting Evidence Into Practice symptom management resources), links to books and articles, continuing education, standards of care
Oncology Section, APTA www.oncologypt.org	Patient resources, oncology fact sheets, and current research

Table 15-3. Examples of Physical Activity and Exercise Resources

Organization	Description
American Tai Chi and Qigong Association www.americantaichi.org/about.asp	Promotes tai chi for public health, physical activity, and overall wellness
Gyrotonic www.gyrotonic.org	Provides individuals with training to teach the Gyrotonic Expansion System method
HEP2Go www.hep2go.com	Provides printable handouts for take-home exercise programs
Jazzercise www.jazzercise.com	Lists franchised organizations that offer aerobic conditioning group classes
National Strength and Conditioning Association www.nsca.com	Offers certification in strength and personal training for special populations
OncoLink www.oncolink.org	Provides information about the benefits of exercise during and after cancer treatment and therapist-created exercise regimens
Pilates Method Alliance www.pilatesmethodalliance.org	Provides individuals with Pilates training and certification
YMCA www.ymca.net	Strengthens the community through lasting personal and social change
Yoga Alliance www.yogaalliance.org	Provides individuals with training and certification to teach yoga
Zumba Fitness www.zumba.com/en-US	Provides individuals with training and licensure to teach Zumba; connects participants with local classes

Summary

Ongoing support for cancer survivors is crucial as they traverse the treatment process and beyond. Adequate support promotes quality of life and opens avenues for socialization. Oncology nurses can help cancer survivors choose appropriate support mechanisms.

References

Beck, S.J., & Keyton, J. (2014). Facilitating social support: Member-leader communication in a breast cancer support group. *Cancer Nursing, 37,* E36–E43. doi:10.1097/NCC.0b013e3182813829

Table 15-4. Outcome Measures for Physical Activity and Exercise

Source	Resources
American Physical Therapy Association http://guidetoptpractice.apta.org	Information on physical therapy interventions as well as common measurements and outcomes
Canadian Society for Exercise Physiology www.csep.ca/en/home	Physical Activity Readiness Questionnaire assessments (PAR-Q and PAR-Q+) (see Chapter 6)
PROQOLID www.proqolid.org	Information on clinical outcome assessments that help patients choose appropriate instruments and facilitate access to them
Rehabilitation Measures Database www.rehabmeasures.org	List of various outcome measures and evidence to support their use in specific populations, including normative values, such as the ones described in Chapter 6

Carr, W., & Wolk, S. (1976). Unmet needs as sociomedical indicators. *International Journal of Health Services, 6,* 417–430.

Gorlick, A., Bantum, E.O., & Owen, J.E. (2014). Internet-based interventions for cancer-related distress: Exploring the experiences of those whose needs are not met. *Psycho-Oncology, 23,* 452–458. doi:10.1002/pon.3443

Hoey, L.M., Ieropoli, S.C., White, V.M., & Jefford, M. (2008). Systematic review of peer-support programs for people with cancer. *Patient Education and Counseling, 70,* 315–337. doi:10.1016/j.pec.2007.11.016

John, D.A., Kawachi, I., Lathan, C.S., & Ayanian, J.Z. (2014). Disparities in perceived unmet need for supportive services among patients with lung cancer in the Cancer Care Outcomes Research and Surveillance Consortium. *Cancer, 12,* 3178–3191. doi:10.1002/cncr.28801

Index

The letter *f* after a page number indicates that relevant content appears in a figure; the letter *t*, in a table.